Intermittent Fasting And The Ketogenic Diet

Shred Fat On The Ultimate Weight Loss Body Transformation Guide For Men And Women (Keto Diet, Healthy Living, Fast Results)

Elliot Cutting

Table of Contents

Intermittent Fasting

Burn Fat And Build Muscle Through Intermittent Fasting For Rapid Weight Loss and a Healthier Lifestyle for Men and Women

Elliot Cutting

Introduction to Intermittent Fasting

Intermittent fasting is a term that refers to a healthy lifestyle trend that is gaining popularity around the world. It involves alternate cycles of eating and fasting. In very simple terms, intermittent fasting involves making a conscious decision to skip one or two meals deliberately.

Dieters follow this lifestyle because of its numerous, proven benefits. These benefits include improved metabolic health, weight loss, longevity, protection against diseases, and a healthy body.

Intermittent fasting is more than just fasting. It is a lifestyle that requires you to take in calories at certain specific times of the day and then consuming absolutely nothing for the remainder of the day.

It's Easy to Lose Fat with Intermittent Fasting

There are plenty of diets out there that people follow. However, more and more health-conscious individuals are choosing intermittent fasting because it works, it is backed by science, it is manageable for the long term, and has numerous health benefits.

1. Calories

A lot of people have misconstrued ideas about why we put on weight. They think it is the choice of food or lack of physical activity. However, according to science, we put on weight because of the consumption of excess calories. Excessive calorie intake is the reason why we put on weight.

By deliberately skipping meals, we reduce our caloric intake on a regular basis. When we reduce the amount of food we eat, then we automatically lose weight. This is the main principle behind intermittent fasting lifestyle and this is why you are still able to eat your favorite foods because your eating window is shortened.

2. Therapeutic

For many centuries, doctors have acknowledged the healing powers of fasting. Since the early 1900s, doctors have successfully used intermittent fasting to address health problems such as diabetes, epilepsy, and obesity.

This approach is now making a successful comeback. Intermittent fasting is now common. Dieters prefer this lifestyle because of its health, weight loss, and therapeutic benefits. By fasting, you get all these healing and therapeutic benefits.

3. Autophagy

One of the most powerful benefits of intermittent fasting is brought about by autophagy. Autophagy is the body's ultimate recycling system. Now, whenever we fast, we set into motion the process of autophagy. When cells in our bodies are deprived of calories, they initiate this process.

Autophagy replaces worn-out and damaged parts of your cells with new ones. This helps to preserve tissue health. Cells in your body create a membrane that hunts down worn-out, diseased, and dead cells and then consumed them. The resulting molecule is then used to create new cell components and to produce energy. In the process, cells also get rid of toxins and consume harmful organism such as those that cause diseases.

Therefore, autophagy performs an effective detoxification throughout the body, helping to eliminate harmful, disease-causing pathogens, eliminating diseased and worn out cells and also reducing inflammation. Normally, autophagy happens when cells in the body digest proteins in order to release amino acids to produce much-needed energy in the body. This process slows down the aging process and promotes metabolism.

What Are the Origins of Fasting?

Fasting simply means deliberate abstinence from drink, food, or both for a specific period of time. It comes in different forms depending on where you live. Absolute fasting is one type. This type of fasting requires total abstinence from all food and drink for a period of about 24 hours.

Man has been fasting for various reasons since time immemorial. Humans and animals naturally resort to fasting during sickness or moments of high stress. Fasting is crucial because it provides rest, balance, and also for energy conservation at critical moments.

Early philosophers, healers, great thinkers, mathematicians, and physicists used fasting as a therapy for healing purposes. Some of these intellectuals include Socrates, Aristotle, Hippocrates, Galen, and Plato. They all spoke favorably about fasting and how therapeutic it is.

Fasting is also common among nearly all major religions of the world. These include Buddhism, Islam, Judaism, and Christianity. Fasting for religious purposes is common among these religions. Faithful fast in order to appeal to a higher deity and sometimes as a form of sacrifice and even cleansing.

Other people and communities fast as part of their traditions. For instance, the Indians of both north and South America fast regularly as they observe certain traditions such as praying for rain or mourning the passing of a great person. Healers of the 19th century used fasting as a form of healing therapy. Yoga practice, which has some fasting elements, has been around for thousands of years. Even ancient healing practices such as Ayurveda include some forms of fasting. Even ordinary people such as you and I practice overnight fasting just about every single day.

Reasons Why People Fast

For religious reasons
Political reasons
Health reasons – to treat an ailment
Medical reasons – for medical procedures, diagnostic purposes

Why is Intermittent Fasting the Easiest Approach?

Research has shown that intermittent fasting is extremely effective when it comes to weight loss – and especially fat loss. It is just as effective as calorie restriction but easier especially compared to other types of diets because of a number of reasons.

1. Intermittent fasting causes insulin levels to drop

When we eat, insulin levels in the body increase. This makes it difficult to lose weight. However, when we fast, insulin levels fall significantly. This allows the body to access fat reserves for energy.

Numerous studies have confirmed that intermittent fasting will not only help to reduce weight but also improve body composition even though results may vary from individual to individual. A study in the 2017 issue of JAMA Internal Medicine shows that dieters stand to lose between 5% and 6% of total body weight when they tried intermittent fasting.

2. Intermittent fasting helps you to retain lean muscle

One of the benefits of losing weight through intermittent fasting is that you only lose fat and not muscle. This is according to Krista Varady, Ph.D., a research scientist at the University of Illinois in Chicago. She is also an associate professor of nutrition and kinesiology at the same institution.

According to her findings, most people who lose weight typically lose 75% fat and 25% muscle mass. However, with intermittent fasting, over 90% of weight loss is fat.

3. You are able to control cravings

One of the reasons why we put on so much weight is because we succumb to cravings. We crave sugar and starch because our bodies are so used to them. Fortunately, when you adopt an intermittent fasting lifestyle, all your cravings will eventually disappear. You will no longer have cravings for unhealthy foods and snacks anymore.

4. Intermittent fasting will drastically reduce cholesterol and triglyceride levels

According to studies recorded in Nutrition Reviews, intermittent fasting has been shown to reduce not just body fat but also triglycerides and cholesterol levels. This is in both overweight and normal weight individuals. This mostly has to do with insulin levels. When you consume fewer calories each day, your blood sugar levels will come down and insulin levels will stabilize.

Is there a catch?

Intermittent fasting is so effective when it comes to weight loss that some people wonder if there is a catch or downside. However, experts agree that there is no real downside to this lifestyle. It is a pretty safe approach to how you eat and live and hardly ever leads to eating disorders.

The only minor challenge that most dieters experience is at the beginning when they have to battle hunger. You can expect the first five days to be challenging because you will feel hungry. However, there are ways to combat hunger pangs. If you are busy, then you mind will most likely not focus on the hunger but on other things.

What makes Intermittent Fasting different from Other Weight Loss Programs?

There are many reasons why intermittent fasting is much better and more effective compared to other diets and weight loss programs. The single most important factor is that intermittent fasting is a lifestyle and not a diet.

Intermittent fasting is a lifestyle that requires you to consciously skip meals occasionally. Most other diets are temporary and have unrealistic goals and requirements. Some are dangerous because of what they require of you. However, intermittent fasting has been proven by health experts, researchers, and others to be effective and manageable in the long run.

Intermittent fasting does not dictate what foods you should eat. What it does is dictate when you should eat and when you should fast. However, to gain the most benefits from this lifestyle, it is advisable to eat natural foods, healthy meals, and nutrients from all major food groups. This way, your body will receive all the essential nutrition it requires from the various food groups.

You can expect to live your best life free from major illnesses and chronic conditions. Since intermittent fasting advocates for a physically active lifestyle, you will enjoy an all-around healthy lifestyle. It also promotes longevity based on numerous studies that have been published.

It is a Diet of Foodies

Sometimes intermittent fasting is referred to as a diet for foodies. A foodie is simply any person who has a keen interest and finer taste for food. Most foodies have gone through a number of diets and the results have not always been pleasant.

If you follow this diet or lifestyle, you will not be limited by food choice. Intermittent fasting actually offers the ultimate flexibility when it comes to food choice. This implies that you are free to enjoy a wide variety of foods even those that are forbidden by other diets and you will still benefit from regular fasts. You will still have to watch your calories but having such a wide variety of foods to choose from is definitely liberating and this makes this lifestyle stand out from the rest.

What Are Doctors Saying About Intermittent Fasting?

Doctors have heard about all the numerous diets and eating patterns out there. They have also read on some of the popular ones like intermittent fasting. However, only intermittent fasting is backed by research and evidence. Most health professionals are impressed with the research findings.

One of the most recent studies, about Cell Metabolism, showcases the benefits of intermittent fasting. The study shows that cutting calories even for short periods of time can bring about serious changes to your body and overall health. However, you should speak to your doctor to ensure that you eat right and do not lose out on important nutrients, especially on fasting days.

Doctors believe this is an excellent lifestyle that, if followed correctly, then it can lead to a healthy lifestyle, weight loss and so much more. Doctors believe that sufficient precaution should be taken. For instance, dieters should not fast for extended periods of time and they should not have any health concerns.

For instance, someone with certain health conditions should generally refrain from partaking in this diet unless with advice from a physician. For instance, pregnant and lactating women, anyone with a history of eating disorders, and those recovering from surgery should refrain from this lifestyle.

Calorie intake is crucial

From the research findings, a lot of the doctors believe it all has to do with calorie intake. The reason is that most dieters who follow this lifestyle follow other diets such as ketogenic, Mediterranean, and so on. When calorie intake is limited, then even overweight and obese individuals will lose weight. Losing weight comes with other benefits such as stable insulin levels, lower blood pressure, better metabolic rate, and also lower cardiovascular risk.

Such a lifestyle should be adapted for the long-term and should not be treated as a fad diet for short-term gain. Diet should not be reduced to an unhealthy cycle of binge eating and calorie restriction because this will defeat the intended purpose. Discipline is necessary and having goals in mind is crucial for long-term success.

Rather than let this lifestyle define you, you should instead focus on good health and getting proper nourishment. When you eat clean, you become healthier and will avoid chronic conditions like heart disease and high blood pressure. Make sure you increase your fruit and vegetable consumption and reduce your carbs intake. If you find a plan that works for you, then you will become mentally and physically healthy and happy.

Chapter 1: Intermittent Fasting Lifestyle

Intermittent fasting lifestyle requires you to adjust your eating habits. When you start following this lifestyle religiously, you will have to deny your body food for a number of hours on particular days.

Intermittent fasting is a lifestyle rather than a diet. You will, therefore, need to be very clear about what you are getting yourself into. Food is usually a big deal in most cultures and our lives revolve around it. As a dieter, you should know that intermittent fasting consists of a number of different protocols. These protocols define fasting and eating times. For instance, we have protocols such as the 5-2 and the 8-6.

The 5-2 protocol dictates normal eating for five days of the week followed by fasting for 2 days of the week. You need to find the intermittent fasting protocol that works for you and suits your regular schedules. For instance, if you are a morning person, then choose a protocol that goes well with mornings.

Also, when choosing your preferred fasting protocol, you should think about the reasons why you are fasting and your regular schedules. Some people are extremely busy during the week but only slightly busy on the weekends. Others wish to lose weight. What you need to do is to ensure that your preferred fasting protocol is in tandem with your lifestyle.

How to Begin the Transition

The transition part is probably going to be your most challenging part. This is because you will start to fast on a regular basis. Your main focus at this time should be to ease into your preferred protocol. You can, for instance, delay your next meal by a couple of hours. If you are in the habit of snacking at midnight, try and cut this out because it is not healthy.

While this lifestyle is majorly about fasting and easing, its success is based on your mental situation. You should train your mind to adjust to this lifestyle. You can, for instance, delay your breakfast by about an hour and then stop your evening meals an hour earlier than usual in order to train the mind of the impending lifestyle changes.

This kind of training of the mind is akin to the way muscles are trained. You first begin training with a lightweight and gradually proceed to increase your weight. This process will continue as you gradually modify your eating habits and general lifestyle.

Getting Started with Intermittent Fasting

One of the main requirements of intermittent fasting is that you change your eating habits. This lifestyle does not necessarily deprive you of food but rather it dictates when you eat and when you fast. Once you begin this lifestyle, then you will have to learn how to go for long stretches without eating.

In most cultures around the world, food is a huge aspect of life and our lives kind of revolve around it. It is crucial that you select the most appropriate protocol so that this new lifestyle works for you. Here are some of the best ways to get started.

o *Choose your preferred fasting protocol*

There are different kinds of protocols that you can follow. They include the 5-2, 16/8, eat-stop-eat, and so on. Think about your lifestyle such as work schedule, family commitments, exercise times, and so on. Find the protocol that best suits your lifestyle.

There are also other factors that you should consider. For instance, what are your reasons for fasting? Most people fast in order to lose weight. If your aim is to lose lots of weight, then you may want to consider the eat-stop-eat or the modified version of the 16-8 protocol where you fast for 18 hours with an eating window of only 6 hours.

○ **Adjust your eating habits**

Plenty of people who start the intermittent fasting lifestyle often consume unhealthy food options. They eat plenty of junk food, processed food, carbonated drinks and so on. The problem with unhealthy eating habits is that they affect your blood sugar, moods, energy levels, and hormones.

You should adjust your diet and start eating clean. Go for healthy, natural foods like vegetables and fruits, whole grains, juices, salads, nuts, and seeds. A healthier diet and regular workouts will result in a healthy body and long-term weight loss.

5 Common Mistakes People Make when Transitioning to Intermittent Fasting

1. Fear of being hungry even for a little while
Feeling hungry is part of life and happens to all of us. In fact, we are hungry a lot of the time. However, being hungry for a couple of hours is generally okay. The hunger pangs will not kill you neither will your strong and lean muscles disappear. This is a fact that has been proven over and over again.

You can lose weight and keep it off while at the same time working out at the gym. Health and fitness expert Jeremy Scott has personal experience when it comes to intermittent fasting. He advises dieters to stick to this lifestyle while lifting weights and generally working out on a regular basis. This way, you will be able to develop lean and strong muscles.

Also, being hungry for a couple of hours will not kill you. Your digestive system will actually benefit from the break. It is very possible to go even 16 to 18 to 24 hours in office. Short-term fasting such as the protocols of intermittent fasting will not cause any significant muscle damage. There are numerous studies that claim that this is actually the case.

2. Eating junk food most of the time

You will not be successful in the long run if you keep eating junk foods, processed foods, fizzy drinks and all that. Experts say that you cannot build a million dollar home on a $1 salary. This statement is absolutely correct.

One of the most common phrases people say is, "I struggle with fat loss." However, you will find that most of the time it has to do with nutrition. Most of the time people do not eat right.

Any person who is struggling with weight loss after adopting the intermittent fasting lifestyle is probably eating the wrong kind of food. Poor quality meals and snacks make it hard to lose weight. Remember that limiting your calorie intake is the best solution to losing weight and keeping it off.

So you need to watch your calorie intake and also ensure that you eat quality calories all the time. This means eating mostly fresh natural foods like fruits and vegetables and avoiding processed foods as much as possible.

3. Jumping into intermittent fasting too fast

One of the reasons why people fail at lifestyle changes and diets is because of jumping in too fast. It is advisable to take a moment and appreciate that intermittent fasting lifestyle is probably completely different from what we are used to.

For instance, if you are used to eating or snacking every two hours and then jump into intermittent fasting, you will find it hard to keep up with the changes. It is advisable to begin slowly and follow protocols such as the 12-12 method. This protocol is ideal for beginners and allows you to fast for 12 hours and then have your meals inside a 12-hour window. A lot of dieters start off this way and many stick to this particular protocol.

4. You eat too much during your eating window
Another very common mistake that beginners make is to eat too much during the eating window. While this lifestyle does not dictate what foods you should eat, common practice dictates that you limit your calorie intake to between 2200 calories for women and 2600 calories for men.

Even if you have been fasting for hours, you still need to watch what you eat. Consuming too many calories during your eating window will constitute excessive calories that will be stored in the body as fat. This will defeat the intended purpose of this otherwise beneficial lifestyle. Sometimes we get so physically and emotionally detached that when the time comes to eat, we overindulge. Therefore, try not to be too preoccupied with your next meal as this is a recipe for disaster.

5. Being too ambitious
Sometimes people start off with extremely high expectations. We notice a friend who has lost plenty of weight due to intermittent lifestyle and decide to jump right in. Some may expect to lose plenty of weight in just a few days. However, you should not be too hard on yourself and do not be too ambitious because the outcome may disappoint you.

Moving from six meals a day to only one meal a day is not only ambitious but rather extreme by any standards. Instead of taking such drastic steps, you should aim for steady but gradual steps until you get used to the new lifestyle. There are other protocols that you can pursue that are pretty effective. Think about the 16-8 protocol or the eat-stop-eat protocol. These are not very taxing and relatively easy to adapt. If you pursue this lifestyle, then you should do so in a structured manner.

Eat your Favorite Foods and Still Lose Weight

Did you know that you can eat your favorite foods and still lose weight? With intermittent fasting, this is very possible. The reason is that intermittent fasting tells you when to eat but not what to eat. Basically, you are not denied your favorite foods. This lifestyle simply advises you when you should eat.

Most of us have a particular food or foods that we cherish. However, sometimes these favorite foods can keep us from losing weight and keeping it off. There are numerous diets out there that deprive us of our favorite foods. Even then, most of these diets do not work or are short-term in nature. Fortunately, intermittent fasting allows you to enjoy your favorite foods while losing weight and leading a healthy lifestyle.

During your fasting period, you should not consume any calories. However, you are allowed to drink water and calorie-free beverages such as black coffee and green tea. During your eating window, you can then have any meal that you like. However, you should watch your calories. This means consuming the recommended amount of calories in order to lose weight or maintain lean muscle. You are supposed to eat clean, healthy, and natural foods most of the time. Therefore if you love meats like steak, chicken, or fish, then you can have these but in moderation.

Intermittent fasting promotes the genes that burn fat and calories. Genes that uncouple proteins and enzymes that are crucial in fat oxidation are activated through fasting. Once these proteins are uncoupled, they produce holes in mitochondria within the body. The mitochondria will then produce less energy because of the holes.

Your body will then be forced to burn more calories in order to produce more energy. Therefore, fasting not only deprives your body of calories but also enhances caloric burn the whole day. When intermittent fasting is done correctly, you may end up eating most of your favorite foods and still lose weight and maintain muscle mass.

Self-Discipline and Intermittent Fasting

If you really want to enjoy the benefits brought about by this lifestyle, then you need to be disciplined. Without discipline, then the lifestyle will probably not work out for you.

One of the most crucial steps is to focus on the benefits of this lifestyle. This will help to keep you motivated. When you feel motivated, then discipline will come automatically.

Discipline means not cheating during fasting. You should not consume any foods or snacks as you fast. Discipline also means avoiding foods that are not good for you such as processed foods, junk foods, and so on. Ensure that you do not consume excessive calories and only eat sufficient amounts of food.

You need to keep in mind that nothing is instant or easy and that everything takes time. Make sure that you keep your mind on your goals and let your desired goals keep you motivated. You should increase your food choice and eat a wide variety. Basically, the wider the variety the better it is for you.

Chapter 2: Types of Fasting

Research findings released in 2017 have shown that intermittent fasting can provide benefits similar to those brought on by calorie restrictions. Calorie restriction has numerous benefits. For instance, it has been proven as the only experimental approach that extends lifespan by 30% and improves the prospects of patients with cancer. However, research has proven that intermittent fasting is more effective compared to calorie restriction.

Health experts such as doctors believe that fasting is actually an excellent idea. It is advisable to starve the body of nutrition a few hours each week a couple of times each week. There is plenty of evidence to showcase the benefits of managed food deprivation. There are different ways of depriving the body of calories. In intermittent fasting, these methods are known as protocols.

There are quite a number of intermittent protocols out there. The choice of protocol by dieters is really a matter of personal preference. There is no one protocol that is better than others. However, some could be more effective than others. You really should find one that fits perfectly with your lifestyle. Some of the common protocols include:

- The 16/8 fasting protocol
- The 5-2 protocol
- Eat-sleep-eat protocol
- The 24-hour fast
- 18/6 fast protocol

The aim of each protocol is to advise you about when to fast and when to eat. However, the basic aim of each protocol is to allow you to fast for a period of time before eventually feasting on purpose. Let us examine these protocols in greater detail.

1. The 16/8 Fasting Protocol

One of the most popular ways of performing intermittent fasting is known as the 16-8 fasting protocols. This protocol requires you to fast for a total of 16 hours within a 24-hour period. You will then have all your meals within an 8-hour window.

As an example, you can have your last meal of the day at 8.00 pm in the night. You will then go to bed at 10.00 pm or 11.00 pm and have nothing to eat until 16 hours later or 12.00 noon the following day. You will then have all your meals and snacks within the next 8 hours or until 8.00 pm the following evening.

You can repeat this cycle as often as you want or follow it a couple of days per week depending on your preferences. This particular protocol has become very popular with dieters around the world especially those seeking to burn fat and lose weight.

While other diet fads and protocols often set out strict regulations and rules, the 16/8 protocol is very simple and easy to follow. It does not place any undue burden on dieters yet it delivers actual results with minimal effort. Apart from enhancing weight loss, this protocol enhances longevity, boosts brain function, and improves blood sugar control.

Positive attributes of the 16/8 fasting protocol

Following this intermittent fasting protocol has been shown to be beneficial to the body in numerous ways all the way to cellular level. Here is a look at some of the benefits associated with this specific fasting protocol.

- o It causes insulin levels in the body to drop to very low levels. This helps the body to burn fat, optimize blood sugar levels and improve the body's insulin sensitivity

- o It results in an increase in the body's levels of HGH or human growth hormone. HGH is a useful hormone that plays a huge role in decreasing body fat and improving the body's composition. The human growth hormone is also extremely useful in matters of cellular regeneration

o   Intermittent fasting protocols such as the 16/8 have been shown to trigger important cellular repair processes like autophagy. Autophagy helps to repair old, worn out, and damaged cells as well as eliminate waste and keep the body healthy

When you follow this protocol, you will be able to fit in between two and four meals within the 8-hour eating window. The 16-8 protocol is also known as the Leangains protocol. You are able to make it a very simple fasting protocol by simply choosing not to have any snacks after dinner and then skipping breakfast the following morning.

Therefore, if your last meal was at 9.00 pm the previous evening, then ensure that you do not have any snacks for the rest of the evening and even the following morning. You will have your next meal the following day at 1.00 pm. You will by this time have fasted for 16 hours straight.

Things to Keep in Mind
Always ensure that you eat mostly healthy foods such as fresh vegetables, lots of fruits, lean meat, whole grains, and so on. The 16/8 protocol is the easiest to follow and also the most natural way of following intermittent fasting. Even as you follow this protocol, ensure that you avoid junk foods and foods that are overly-processed as these are not good for your body.

2. The 5-2 Fast Diet Protocol

The other protocol that is popular with intermittent fasting is the 5–2 protocol which is also known as the fast diet. There are those who believe that this particular protocol is the most popular of all intermittent fasting protocols. One reason why it is so popular is because it allows you to eat normally for five days of the week and then you get to fast for only two days of the week.

The fasting days should be non-consecutive rather than consecutive. Therefore you will have to restrict your calorie intake for two non-consecutive by limiting your meals to a total of 500 – 600 calories per day.

A lot of dieters find this particular protocol easy to follow and easier to adapt compared to others. And since you do not have to fast each and every single day, this protocol is considered more of a lifestyle than a diet. It does not dictate any foods that you should or should not eat but only when to fast and when to eat.

500 – 600 Calories

During your fast days, you will consume a total of 500 calories for women and 600 calories for men. You will fast for most of the day and then only eat during your 8-hour eating window. For the remainder of the week, you are allowed to eat normally and have regular meals.

5-2 Protocol for Weight Loss

One of the benefits of this protocol is that it is effective for weight loss. If you follow it correctly, then you will lose weight and body fat. This is because this diet requires you to limit your calorie intake not just on your fasting days but even on days when you don't fast. It is important therefore that you do not over-indulge on your non-fast days.

If you follow this diet as recommended, then you should expect to lose between 3% and 8% of your body weight within 3 to 24 weeks. This is according to a study published here in this scientific journal. This study shows that properly abiding by the 5-2 protocol will help you lose anywhere between 4% and 8% of your waist circumference. This means losing large amounts of dangerous belly fat.

Eating on Your Fast Days

There is generally no guiding rule on how to eat on your fast days. Some people prefer eating nothing all day and then have their meals during the small eating window. Others prefer having a small breakfast and then a meal much later in the evening. What you need to keep in mind is that you should eat a maximum of 500 calories for women and 600 calories for men. It is advisable, as such, to plan your meals accordingly. Ensure that your meals are healthy, full of fiber, and sufficient nutrition. High protein, low-glycemic carbs, vegetables, and fruits are highly recommended. These foods are not only highly nutritious but will also keep you feeling full for longer.

3. Alternate-Day Fasting

Another intermittent fasting protocol that is out there is the alternate-day protocol. This protocol requires you to fast every other day. This means you will alternate between fast days and normal eating days. You can modify this protocol to eat a maximum of 500 calories on your fast days and about 2200 – 2600 on non-fast days.

This particular protocol is very popular and effective for weight loss. It also comes with numerous other benefits. Your eating is only restricted half of the time but the benefits that you receive are immense. You can drink as much water and non-caloric beverages as you like. Non-caloric beverages include green tea, black coffee, and unsweetened tea. You should avoid all other types of drinks especially those sugary drinks, sodas, and carbonated drinks. These are not good for your body. This protocol allows you to consume between 20% and 25% of your energy requirements which totals to about 500 calories.

Studies done by nutrition scientists at the University of Chicago show that those who follow intermittent fasting can lose as much as 8% of their body weight in 3 to 12 weeks. This lifestyle is particularly useful for women as well especially those aged between 40 to 60 years. It helps to reduce stubborn belly fat and the results are far more impressive compared to traditional weight loss methods. Intermittent fasting is the number one choice for numerous dieters because it is easy to follow, has very few restrictions, is very effective and with amazing outcomes.

4. The 24-Hour Fast Protocol

Yet another method of following the intermittent fasting is the 24-hour protocol. This protocol requires you to fast for a 24-hour period or an entire day. For instance, if you have your last meal tonight at 8.00 pm, then you will eat nothing for the next 24 hours until 8.00 pm the following evening. However, you do not have to adhere to this protocol each and every day or even every other day. You can instead choose to apply it once or twice a week.

One reason why some prefer this protocol is because of issues to do with impulse eating or binge eating. People tend to eat when they feel lonely, excited, frustrated, happy, confused, or stressed. This means the food is used to address our emotional situation. Using food as a response to emotions does not provide the best approach to these issues. Feeding emotional hunger instead of real hunger is definitely not acceptable.

This particular fast enables you to differentiate between emotional and actual hunger. If you learn how to do without food even when stressed or emotional, then you will eventually learn how to cope with your emotions without then need for food.

In some cases, you may be unable to go without food for an entire 24-hour period. Fortunately, intermittent fasting is a flexible lifestyle that allows you to make acceptable adjustments. For instance, if you are unable to fast for an entire 24-hour period, then it is okay to fast for 22, 20, or even 18 hours. In short, you should not give up hope if things do not quite work out the first time. Just do the best that you can and keep improving on that.

Spontaneous and Convenient Meal Skipping

Apart from the above protocols, there are other flexible forms of intermittent fasting that are widely accepted. Remember that the aim of this lifestyle is to go for long stretches of time without having anything to eat. One such protocol allows you to skip a meal whenever it is convenient to do so. There is no protocol to follow or rules to adhere with. All you simply do is skip a meal whenever possible and stand to see the results thereafter.

You can choose to skip a meal whenever you are busy or not feeling very hungry. There have been previous misconceptions about having to eat so many meals each day. However, this is not always the case and you can skip meals occasionally. You will suffer no harm if you skip a meal yet you stand to enjoy certain benefits.

The human body is aptly designed to handle stress including hunger. Meal skipping is not a stressful form of fasting but rather a convenient one that can be adapted from time to time. Even this simple approach has some health benefits to you so try and see where you fit best with these different fasting protocols.

The 16/8 Protocol is Highly Recommended

If you want to adopt the intermittent fasting lifestyle, then you should opt for the 16/8 protocol. This is the model practiced successfully by most dieters. You are likely to succeed following this protocol compared to others especially if you wish to lose weight and keep it off. For long-term health and wellness, the 16/8 protocol offers you the best chance for success.

Chapter 3: Transitioning to Intermittent Fasting

Intermittent fasting requires you to change your meal times so that you stay for lengthy periods of time without eating. This lifestyle offers you an excellent opportunity to lose body fat, weight, and maintain lean muscle. It will enable you to drastically shed pounds by cutting down calorie intake without going on any crazy diets. In fact, it is possible to keep your normal calorie intake while still following this lifestyle.

Getting Started with Intermittent Fasting

One of the things that you need to do is to adjust your eating habits. You will not be depriving your body of food or nutrition. Instead, you will be eating much later or earlier than usual. This lifestyle simply requires you to deny yourself food and nourishment for a couple of hours during the day or night.

While this process can seem daunting at first, what you need to do is to approach it using the following steps.

- o Breakdown the fasting process into small yet simple, doable steps
- o Simple step-by-step actions will guarantee success
- o Make observations at each stage then analyze the observation
- o Come up with a conclusion about the observation and analysis

However, before you get started, there are a couple of things that you need to. You should first speak with a healthcare expert such as a doctor.

1. Speak to a doctor before starting: It is absolutely important to speak to your physician about this lifestyle before you begin. Your doctor will assess your health and advice about any medical condition you may have. Generally, if you are pregnant, are lactating, have a chronic condition or other issues of concern, then your doctor will advise you appropriately.

2. Keep it simple: It is advisable to keep things as simple as possible. When you fast, you are allowed to take water, black coffee, unsweetened tea, or green tea.

3. Take it easy: Try and eat your normal meals when you are not fasting. For best outcomes, try and focus on low carb diets, whole foods, fruits, and vegetables. Also, remember to stay hydrated. At this juncture, you will want to launch a program that has great chances of success. Your goal really should be to get to the end of your fast successfully.

4. Time: Do not be too blinded by days or time. These are provided only as a guide. For instance, you do not have to start or complete your fasts at a fixed time, say 10.00 am or 2.00 pm. You can choose to follow indicated times but generally, you should set times and choose days that best suit you and your lifestyle.

5. Best day of the week: It is up to you to choose which days of the week that you will fast. Fasting on weekdays is more convenient compared to weekends because these are structured. Most people prefer to fast on Mondays, Wednesdays, or Thursdays. Try not to fast on consecutive days.

6. Slip-ups are fine: Sometimes we fail in our quests to follow this lifestyle. If you forget to fast or consume too many calories, do not despair. Some people are prone to giving in. basically, just do what you need to do and then get back on track.

Additional steps to get you started

1. Determine what your fasting goal is

You need to first determine what your fasting goals are. What is the purpose you wish to achieve through intermittent fasting? For some, it could be weight loss and weight maintenance. Fasting has been proven to reduce some hormones such as insulin while increasing others like HGH or the human growth hormone and norepinephrine.

You can decide to fast in order to relieve symptoms of a certain illness or even to avoid medication. Fasting can help you to better manage chronic conditions such as heart disease and diabetes and even internal inflammation. It is great for preventing serious diseases while increasing longevity.

2. Address all your fears and worries

It is common to have concerns, questions, and worries, especially when embarking on a journey. It is also possible that there are aspects of intermittent fasting that bother you. If so, then you should address all these fears, as answers are available to them all.

Can I skip breakfast? Absolutely, you really don't have to have breakfast and it is not the most important meal of the day. Numerous dieters view it as a neutral meal which won't affect your life much. For instance, it will not cause you to lose weight nor will it fire up your metabolism.

Should I avoid snacks? If you wish to skip snacks then that is okay. Snacking is generally allowed as part of intermittent fasting but not snacking is also okay. It is a habit that won't cause you to lose weight, as it does not boost metabolism. However, unplanned snacking can contribute to liver disease and obesity. Metabolism will not slow down. It is a known fact that fasting does increase your metabolism. When your metabolism rate increases, then you will increase and retain your muscle mass even as you lose weight.

Other Crucial Considerations

o *Choose your preferred fasting protocol*

There are a number of different fasting protocols out there. Study them closely and see which ones are the most suitable for your lifestyle. It will be much easier for you if you get a protocol that is in tune with your lifestyle.

For example, if you are more of a morning person who enjoys working hard in the morning and enjoying a snack thereafter, then identify the protocol that is close to this lifestyle. Others love to work out in the evening so find which one will generally match your lifestyle.

If you choose to fast two days a week, then choose days such as Mondays and Wednesdays or Tuesdays and Thursdays. This way, you will be able to fast with little distraction compared to fasting over the weekend when there are parties, visits, family members and so on.

You can choose the eat-stop-eat protocol in this instance. This means that on your fasting days, you will fast for 16 hours each day and then have all your meals and snacks within the 8-hour eating window. You will mostly consume not more than 500 calories for women and 600 calories for men on your fasting days. On other days, you will aim for 2200 – 2400 for women and 2400 – 2600 for men on your other days.

There are a couple of other factors that you will need to consider when choosing your preferred protocol. For instance, are you trying to lose weight, fast for the long term, or for religious reasons? If you can answer these questions, then you will be able to clearly choose the most appropriate protocol that is aligned with your lifestyle. You will be more flexible if your reasons for fasting include anti-aging, building lean muscle or longevity and so on.

- ○ *Adjust your eating habits*

You should start considering adjusting your eating habits at this stage. The attractive aspect of intermittent fasting is the fact that it does not dictate what foods to eat but rather when to eat and when to fast.

However, you should choose healthy, natural foods rather than junk food or highly processed foods. A healthy diet and occasional workouts are necessary for weight loss and a healthy body. Unhealthy foods such as junk food will leave you feeling lethargic and will not support your weight loss ambitions.

- ○ *Conduct sufficient research all the time*

Intermittent fasting has numerous health benefits. However, it has a number of protocols. You need to identify one of these protocols and then make a determination about it. You should really be guided by your lifestyle when choosing a particular protocol to follow.

Now Begin the Transition

Now that you have a lot of relevant information, you should begin intermittent fasting. Ensure that you ease gently into your preferred protocol. You may find that it involves delaying your first of the day as much as possible. You should avoid late night eating or snacking.

Hydration is Crucial as You Fast

You need to stay hydrated as you fast. Water is crucial for the body and a major necessity for numerous processes. You need to stay hydrated so that normal processes proceed without a hitch.

Water hydrates the body. It also plays other crucial roles. For instance, it is used to eliminate toxins from the body and this is why some experts believe that you should drink plenty of water even as you fast. Some say that you should drink at least 8 glasses each day.

On top of frequent water drinking, you need to take plenty of other beverages. These include unsweetened tea, green tea, and black coffee. These beverages help to keep you hydrated as well as fight off hunger pangs.

Remember to spread your hydration throughout the day. If you drink too much water all at once, you will not hydrate properly as you will eliminate most of it almost immediately.

How to Overcome Hunger Pangs

If you wish to overcome hunger pangs as you fast, then you need to make deliberate stops to avoid feeling hungry. Hunger can be both physiological and physical. If you manage to conquer hunger especially in the early days, then you will be alright.

1. Ensure that you have the right mindset: you need to understand and appreciate that fasting is real and that you are likely to feel hungry especially at the onset. You need to keep in mind that you are not likely to suffer any setbacks because of fasting. If you start feeling hungry just at the onset of fasting, then you should not give in and think that it is not possible. Instead, you should hold out for as long as you can. Also, you should not be fantasizing about your next meal or snack. Instead, you should keep busy and focus on your work and other things. You should also think about all the benefits you stand to gain by fasting regularly.

2. Understand that there is real hunger and psychological hunger. There are two distinct types of hunger. There is the general hunger that we feel after abstaining from food for a long period of time. Physical hunger can be satiated with food. However, you may also suffer from psychological hunger. Emotional or psychological hunger is different. It results from many causes such as stress, emotional pain, guilt, worry, and so on. Psychological hunger keeps you craving for more and more food especially the processed kind. You usually feel uncomfortably full after eating and this makes you feel guilty.

3. Keep both your mind and body active: Being active is crucial as it keeps your mind focused elsewhere. If you are not busy then you will focus on the hunger pains and keep thinking about food. Therefore, try and focus on things other than food. For instance, if you are employed, then try and focus on the work at hand. You should immerse yourself in activities even when you are not working. When you are generally busy and with constant flow, then you will notice that time flies very fast. Being busy also helps you to lose weight.

4. Take a tablespoon or two of Psyllium Husk: Psyllium Husk is an edible type of soluble fiber and has numerous benefits for the body. It also serves as a prebiotic which is excellent for the digestive system. This is why it is often used as a dietary supplement. When you take this product regularly or as advised, it will draw water from your colon and sweep it clean of all waste. You will stop feeling full or bloated. Psyllium is known to promote a healthy heart and it has a positive effect on cholesterol levels.

5. Battling hunger as you fast: As you progress along your intermittent fasting journey, you will note that hunger is only a problem during the initial stages. As soon as your body begins to get used to the change, it will be easier for you to cope. You should expect to suffer serious hunger pangs for the first two to three weeks. After the fourth week, hunger will cease to be a major issue.

Things You Need to Unlearn

Research conducted by various institutions has opened our eyes to certain truths. There is a lot of misinformation out there. A lot of people currently have the wrong misinformation about calorie intake, type of foods to eat, and so much more. Here are a couple of things that we need to unlearn.

1. We need to eat six small meals per day spread throughout the day

There was a time that people strongly believed in having six complete meals each day. These include breakfast, tea, lunch, a snack, dinner, and dessert. We all thought that this is how we ought to live. Fortunately, we have now learned through research that we can survive without snacks. We can also survive on 2 to 3 meals per day.

2. Fasting can cause you serious harm

There is a popular belief that claims fasting or nutrition deprivation can have serious health consequences even after a short while. Well, we now know differently. Fasting is common among many communities around the world. It has been practiced for centuries with excellent results. The truth is that fasting will not do you any harm but it will help you overcome many challenges you may be facing. Fasting can help you combat diseases, illnesses and also keep you looking young and healthy.

3. Breakfast is the most crucial meal of the day

We have for a long time been of the opinion that breakfast is essential and must be had each morning. This has now been established to be false. We do not need to have breakfast at all. It is an optional meal that we can do without. Breakfast is also not the most crucial meal of the day. You can, therefore, choose whether to have breakfast or skip it regularly.

4. Late night eating is bad for you

For a long time, we have been told not to eat late in the night. Many people believe that late night eating will make you fat and cause you to add weight. The reasoning is that the calories from your late-night meal or midnight snack will be stored as fat as you do not engage in any activities as you sleep. However, that is not how it works. The body does not care what time you eat. What matters is the total number of calories consumed. Therefore, do not be too concerned about when you eat but rather the total number of calories per day.

5. All fats are bad for you

Fats, together with carbs, have long been castigated as bad for the body. People generally believe that fats are not healthy and are bad for you. They are stored all over the body and are thought to clog the arteries. It is true that saturated fats and trans fats are bad for you. They are the ones found in packaged foods and snacks and can negatively affect your health and weight.

However, monounsaturated and polyunsaturated fats are actually really good for the body when taken in moderation. These oils are found in nuts, olives, fatty fish, and avocados. They are good for your heart and brain and great for the skin. They are absolutely essential for any healthy diet and are great for your health too. It is therefore quite okay to enjoy a healthy dose of fatty foods every day just as long as these are monounsaturated and polyunsaturated fats.

Intermittent Fasting and Exercise

If you truly want to reap the maximum benefits from the fasting lifestyle, then you should ensure that you engage in regular exercises and workouts. For effective exercises, you should consider coming up with a work out regime. However, things can get tricky when you are fasting because of energy levels. You will need to take some precautions if you are to exercise in a fasted state. Here are a couple of things that you can consider.

1. Plan your meals around your workouts

If you want to lose a lot of weight very fast, then you may want to do is workout on an empty stomach. What this means is that you will work out before having anything to eat. This can be tricky at first so you should plan your meals accordingly. However, it is a very effective weight loss plan.

You can wake up in the morning and probably go for a jog, a swim, or do some cardio workouts. However, you should ensure that you eat the right kind of foods the night before. For instance, you should have some complex carbs and protein. These will help you build your glycogen stores with the right kind of energy. If you do this you will have sufficient energy for your workouts.

Try never to work out on a full stomach. All you need to ensure that you do is to plan early, think about your workouts and what time you wish to work out. The crucial point that you need to note is that your nutrition needs should match the demands of your workouts even when you have to work out early in the morning.

2. Use the best approach

Basically, whenever you work out, you should do so to your heart's content. However, you should stop if you start feeling dizzy, lightheadedness or sick. This can occur whenever you are fasting. Things will get easier once you get used to fasting. Try and start out with less taxing workouts and light exercises especially if you are not used to fasting. If you do so, then your blood sugar levels will drop to serious levels and you may start feeling dizzy.

Remember to pay attention to your body and listen to what it says. If you feel sick or weak, stop and take a break. You can always work out at a different time. Also, a little planning goes a long so always remember to plan ahead and prepare adequately before your workouts.

Things that You are Allowed to Have

1. Black Coffee

You are allowed to drink Black coffee as you fast. Having this in your fasted state helps to reduce appetite and stave off hunger. Coffee also accelerates metabolism and has a positive effect on your strength and stamina.

If you don't like Black coffee and alternative can be Zero sugar energy drinks that have no calories. This is not recommended however if you need a kick of energy during your fast, this is an alternative.

2. Water

You should take plenty of water. Water is essential as it performs important functions in the body. It is funny though because most people forget to drink sufficient amounts of water yet this is a simple requirement. people avoid drinking water because it has a flat taste and keeps sending them to the bathroom. However, water flushes toxins from your body and leaves you well hydrated. It also keeps you feeling full and you do not have to worry about feeling hungry.

3. Green tea

If you do not like the taste of water, then you can add a slice of lemon to improve the taste. Lemon does not just improve the taste of water but also helps to kill off germs in your system. Alternatively, you can opt for green tea.

Apparently, green tea is excellent for you even as you fast. Green tea dramatically reduces hunger pangs and enables you to stay focused on the task ahead rather than your next meal. Green tea contains catechins which are effective in burning fat, especially stubborn tummy fat.

Green tea also contains powerful antioxidants that help with detoxification. It supports autophagy which is the body's own cleansing mechanism. Green tea also helps to eliminate free radicals which are very harmful to the body. Therefore, always have a cup of green tea handy as you fast.

Bone broth? There are suggestions that bone broth is ideal when you are fasting. Bone broth contains very few calories but is excellent in your fasted state. It contains some micronutrients that provide you with energy. If you get to feel very hungry, then you should warm a cup and have it in your fasted state.

Chapter 4: Counting Your Calorie Intake

What are Macronutrients?

Macronutrients can be defined as nutrients that provide the body with energy or calories. Nutrients are chemicals or substances that are essential for certain functions in the body such as metabolism and growth.

Macronutrients are needed in large amounts and this is why we use the term "macro". Macro means large or huge. There are three major macronutrients that are essential to humans. These are;

- ○ Lipids
- ○ Proteins
- ○ Carbohydrates

There are certain quantities of calories that we receive when we eat foods from each group. Carbohydrates and proteins provide 4 calories per gram while fat provides 9 calories per gram. Alcohol provides 7 calories per gram. However, it is not a macronutrient and is not essential for life.

Humans need macronutrients, water, and micronutrients for survival. Micronutrients are essential nutrients that our bodies required in smaller amounts. They include minerals and vitamins.

Proteins: We need to consume proteins each and every day. According to health recommendations, we need to ensure that between 10% and 35% of all the calories that we consume. All human cells contain protein and it constitutes a major part of our organs, muscles, glands, muscles, and the skin.

Carbohydrates: according to science, our bodies need carbohydrates in the largest amount compared to other macronutrients. Of all the calories we consume daily, about 45% to 65% should be from carbohydrates. There are a number of reasons why carbohydrates are so crucial. Here are those reasons.

- Carbohydrates are the body's most crucial source of energy
- They are easily absorbed by the body
- Are crucial for waste elimination and intestinal health
- Are easily stored in the liver and muscles for future energy use
- Are essential in muscles, brain, kidneys, nervous system, heart

Almost all living organisms, both animals and plants, do contain some carbohydrates. Even then, it is easier to obtain them from some sources compared to others. For instance, starches are a great source of carbohydrates. Examples of starches are;

- Cereal grains such as rice, barley, wheat, millet, and oats
  Fruits like bananas, grapes, plums, cherries, dates, apricots,   melons, apples, etc.
- Legumes such as peas, lentils, beans, and peanuts
  Starchy vegetables such as pumpkin, yams, cassava root,   potatoes, etc.
- Mildly starchy veggies such as cauliflower, beets, carrots, salsify

Fats: A lot of people have negative thoughts about fats and fatty oils. This is because they are blamed for weight gain. However, fats are essential for human survival. The recommended daily fat intake is 20% to 33% of all the calories that you consume.

Fat consists of individual fatty acids. These fatty acids are generally the building blocks that fats are made of. Some of the most useful fatty acids in the body are omega-3 and omega-6.

These are also known as essential fatty acids. They are important mainly for two reasons mostly. They are used in the production of substances that control chemical reactions in the cells and also help in the formation of cell membranes or outer layer of cells. Fats are essential for the following purposes;

- They provide organs with cushioning
- Are essential for normal growth and development
- Fats are needed for absorption of fat-soluble vitamins
- Are an excellent source of energy
- They make food stable, consistent, and tasty
- They help to maintain cell membranes

Fiber: This is a carbohydrate that is not digested by the body. This carbohydrate passes through the alimentary canal and aids in waste elimination. It is advisable to consume foods that are high in fiber as they have been shown to reduce the risks of obesity and high disease. They have also been proven to lower high cholesterol. Such foods include whole grains, vegetables, and fruits.

Putting this information to use

- Bake or grill your food rather than fry it
- Choose smoked mackerel instead of some greasy fry-up
- Always choose lean meat such as fish and chicken over steaks
- Choose sauces made out of tomatoes
- Grate cheese if you have to so as to make it last longer

When you work so hard and watch what you eat in order to lose weight, you probably assume others have the same knowledge. If you don't then you could possibly be fumbling in the dark. Some of the most crucial steps you will need to follow include working out more and learning how to count calories and use a food tracker.

Calories do not represent nutrition but energy

When you fill your plate with food, it is only the calories do not give a full picture of what's going on but just part of it. Calories are an indicator of the amount of energy that you eat. However, they do not paint a full picture of the quality or nutrition that you take.

When you count calories, you are able to receive the correct amount of energy that your body needs and also ensure that you work towards your weight loss goals.

Counting Macronutrients

All the food that we eat consists of three macros. These are protein, carbohydrates, and fats. They are the building blocks of the food we eat. There is a difference, however, between tracking macros and counting calories. If you only count macros then you could lose out on crucial nutrients.

Tracking macros

Tracking macros encourage a healthier choice of food types. When you track your macros, you will be able to determine the quality of your calories. You will ensure that your foods come from all the three major sources of calories. Tracking macros are good for you. There are rations available that have been determined by nutrition bodies such as the Food and Nutrition Board of the IOM or institution of Medicine.

If you want to eat healthy as per the recommendations of the Food and Nutrition Board, then you should aim to have 20 – 35% of your diet in the form of fats, 10 – 35% proteins, and 45% - 65% carbs. I recommend going low carbs and high fats and proteins if you want to lose more fat and build more muscle.

How to Track Macronutrients

It is crucial that you learn how to track the macronutrients – proteins, carbohydrates, and fats. By tracking these important nutrients, you will be able to consume a well-balanced diet on a regular basis and also attain your specific dietary goals.

Counting macronutrients, especially for homemade meals is pretty simple. You will need to follow a step-by-step procedure in order to attain your goals. All you need to do to successfully work out your macronutrient intake is to answer two questions. You will need to be able to break down your food to the macronutrient level and then determine how much of it you want to eat.

1. Identify the different food items in your meal

If your meal comes packaged with a label, then you can skip this step. However, if you prepared the meal from scratch at home, then you will need to make a note of each item in the meal. Get a piece of paper or even a tabulated sheet such as an Excel or Google sheet. Your meal could, for instance, include zucchini, onions, tomatoes, garlic, and some extra virgin olive oil. List all these food items down.

2. Calculate the quantity of each food serving for those with labels

If you purchase pre-packed food, then you should be able to see the serving sizes. Simply take the quantity that you consumed and divide this by the serving size. Once you get the answer, you will then determine the individual macronutrients in the food in order to determine how much of each you ate.

3. Make use of the USDA Food Search tool

Use the chart described to determine the levels of calories in your food. Fresh fruits and vegetables are often referred to as "raw foods" as they are unprocessed. You can also use the search tool to determine the quantity that best represents the amount of each macronutrient on your plate.

Once you are able to break down your food into macros and then determine the amount of each on your plate, you will be able to work out the calorie content of each. Using the Food Search tool is pretty easy if you have the right information.

Now sum up all the protein in your plate, all the carbohydrates, and all the fats. You will find figures or values such as total protein = 48.6 grams, total carbohydrates = 238.4 grams and total fats = 62.6 grams. Now you need to convert these figures into calories. This is pretty simple because we already know the amount of calories in each macronutrient.

Use a food tracker application program or App

Alternatively, you can use a food tracker app. If you find that tracking macronutrients are a little challenging, then you can use an application program or app. Rather than calculating your TDEE or total daily energy expenditure, you can use a health tracker to work this out for you.

Using a food tracker helps to save you time, eliminates any guesswork, and provides you with more detailed figures than you need. Some of these apps have macro-based meal plans so that you do not have to be concerned about how to increase carbohydrate levels while keeping other macronutrients the same.

Calculating Macros for Weight Loss

In order to work out the necessary macros for weight loss, you need to determine your TDEE or total daily energy expenditure. This is simply the total amount of calories or energy that you expend each day. If you want to lose weight, you will eat less and less food each day.

There is a basic formula used to calculate your TDEE. In fact, there are plenty of formulae. However, the most important one used today is known as the Mifflin St. Jeor formula.

Resting energy expenditure (REE): This is the energy that your body uses when you are resting.

Males: REE = 10 X weight (kg) + 6.25 X height (cm) – 5X age(yrs) + 5

Females: REE = 10 X weight (kg) + 6.25 X height (cm) – 5X age (yrs) – 161

However, most people do not just sit down all day. They engage in one activity or the other. Therefore, once you work out the REE, you can then determine the TDEE of individuals based on their physical activity.

Sedentary lifestyle: TDEE = REE X 1.2
Light activity: TDEE = REE X 1.375
Moderate activity: TDEE = REE X 1.55
Very active: TDEE = REE X 1.725

An example of how to work out your calories
Let us assume that you are a 30-year-old man weighing 80kg, 184 cm, who is moderately active. This is the equation that will determine how much calories you consume each day.

[10 X weight (kg) + 6.25 x height (cm)] – [5 X age (yrs) + 5 = REE] X 1.55

(10 X 80) + (6.25 X 184) – (5 X 30) + 5 = REE
800 + 1150 – 150 + 5 = 1805

Since you are moderately active, we will multiply the REE X 1.55 = 2797 calories

Therefore, based on your activity level and body measurements, you will consume about 2797 calories per day. For weight loss purposes, you should shed your calories by not more than 20%. For weight maintenance, eat calories equivalent to your TDEE. However, if you eat more calories than this, then you will definitely gain weight.

Tracking your Macros

If you wish to track your calories, then experts advise that you use a suitable app or application program. There are plenty of reliable ones out there. One that comes highly recommended is known as MyFitnessApp. It is available on both Android and iOS platforms. You can also use the MyMacros+ which is even more flexible and has a lot more variables and options for you.

Alternatively, you can buy and use a food scale. While plenty of nutritional information is available on food packaging, you can still use a food scale which is a lot more accurate. Using a food scale will ensure that you are accurately tracking the food that you eat.

Best Time to Work Out when Fasting

There are no specific work out times because people have different preferences. However, it has been shown that working out early in the morning on an empty stomach is the best for weight loss. Even health experts recommend working out on an empty stomach.

You can go for an early morning jog or gym work out. If you plan to work out in the morning, and then ensure that you eat a suitable dinner the night before. Complex carbohydrates should be part of your dinner because they release energy slowly.

Then we have fasted workouts or fasted cardio. This is when you work out during your fasting period. It is one of the best approaches for anyone looking to lose weight. However, you need to be careful whenever you opt for fasted cardio. Your body can be depleted of energy reserves and this will leave you feeling weak and dizzy. It is advisable to avoid fasted workouts until your body gets used to the fasting lifestyle.

Chapter 5: Health Benefits of Intermittent Fasting

There are numerous health benefits of intermittent fasting. These include physical benefits, mental, and physiological. It is a fact that what is good for the body is also good for your brain as well. While on the major benefits of intermittent fasting is weight loss, there are plenty of other benefits throughout the body.

Intermittent fasting not only helps with weight loss but also helps to improve certain metabolic features that are great for the brain. These include lower insulin resistance and reduced blood sugar levels, reduced inflammation and lower levels of oxidative stress.

To understand the benefits of intermittent fasting, it is important to also appreciate what happens to the body when we fast especially at cellular level. When you fast, your body does not have all the food it needs to produce energy. However, the body must have energy. Therefore, the liver begins breaking down amino acids and fats into glucose. Your energy levels will reduce as the body begins conserving energy.

A process known as ketosis will begin. At this stage, the body will begin to burn stored fats to produce energy. As soon as it sets in, you will then stop feeling hungry or lightheadedness. At the same time, your blood pressure will fall and the heart rate will slow down. Ketosis is excellent for balancing blood sugar and promoting weight loss and other physiological benefits.

Evidence-Based Benefits of Intermittent Fasting

1. You lose weight and stubborn belly fat

One of the major benefits of intermittent fasting is that you lose weight and shed off the pounds. This is because the body will stop relying on food to produce energy as you fast and instead reach into fat reserves. Therefore, when you start fasting, you begin a slow but steady weight loss process. As you keep this lifestyle up, you will notice further weight loss. Expect to lose anywhere between 3% and 8% of your total body weight in just 3 to 24 weeks.

2. It supports the regulation of functions of genes, hormones, and cells

There is clear research-based evidence showing that intermittent fasting regulates hormones in the body and also ensures superior hormonal balance. As you fast, the organs get to rest and this includes the liver which is a crucial organ necessary for balancing hormones.

Insulin: this is a hormone that is released by the pancreas. Its function is to regulate the sugar levels in the blood. As you fast, the body starts converting stored fats into energy in order to fuel cell activity. As the body loses more fat, it becomes more responsive to insulin and it gets absorbed more.

Better absorption of insulin in the body results in better blood sugar regulation. This helps to prevent diabetes or manage it such that sometimes patients may not need to use medication. Thus intermittent fasting offers an excellent solution that helps prevent diabetes. Insulin resistance is a situation that occurs due to excessive glucose in the blood.

Human growth hormone: HGH or human growth hormone is responsible for multiplication and division of cells. It also promotes and stimulates the synthesis of collagen in skeletal muscles and tendons. HGH improves your physical performance and boosts your immune system. Fasting boosts HGH levels in the blood by almost 5 times. It has numerous benefits to the body including the development of strong bones, lean muscle, healthy hair growth and so much more.

Cortisol: It is also known as the stress hormone. It is supplied to the body when it is stressed. This is why it is also known as the fight or flight hormone. It triggers just that kind of response. This stress hormone is properly regulated by regular fasting. When insulin is properly managed, very little cortisol is released into the body.

Estrogen: The female hormone estrogen can cause issues such as weight gain, irritability, and headaches if it is present in large numbers. An enzyme known as aromatase, found in most tissues, converts testosterone into estrogen. This enzyme is prevalent in fatty cells so individuals with high-fat levels usually have elevated estrogen levels. Low-fat levels in the body reduce the presence of aromatase and in return estrogen levels will reduce.

Cells: Cells provide storage space for fats and sometimes dangerous pathogens. During fasting sessions, your body reaches out the cells and utilizes the stored fat. In the process, the body also consumes or eliminates all pathogens found in such cells. Also, the cells get renewed and rejuvenated with newer cells produced that are more efficient, fat-free, effective, and efficient.

3. Intermittent fasting enhances metabolism
When you fast, you provide the digestive system with relief. Regular fasting tends to boost metabolism which ensures that the body burns fat more efficiently. Fasting combined with regular exercises provide the best way of losing weight, shedding fat and keeping it off, becoming fit and so on. Intermittent fasting enhances metabolism by cleansing the cells on the inside. It also helps to regulate your digestive system and metabolic action. In the process, it also promotes healthy bowel function and also improves the metabolic action.

The minute that your metabolism slows down, the aging process will begin. This is why an efficient metabolism keeps aging at bay. Fasting provides your digestive system a break from the usual grind of digestion. Again, when you improve your eating habits by eating the right foods in the right quantity, you will energize your metabolism so that it becomes efficient and functions as required.

4. It reduces the risk of type II diabetes

One of the most serious chronic conditions is type II diabetes. It is a condition or disease that occurs due to excessive amounts of blood sugar in the body. Our bodies usually produce insulin in order to help regulate blood sugar levels. However, levels of blood sugar can increase greatly such that the insulin levels cannot manage it. Diabetes is usually the result of excessive blood sugar levels that cannot be managed. When the body becomes resistant to insulin, then glucose will accumulate in tissues not designed for fat storage.

Intermittent fasting has been proven to reduce blood sugar levels and keep them down to manageable levels for the short, medium, and long terms. With fasting comes a drastic reduction of blood sugar levels as well as excessive fats. You can expect a reduction in blood sugar levels of between 3% and 6% once you start fasting. Therefore, fasting can have a major and positive effect on blood sugar levels.

5. Intermittent fasting boosts your immune system

One of the crucial systems in the body is the immune system. It provides you with protection against dangerous pathogens, diseases, and infections of all kinds. According to research by scientists at the University of Southern California, fasting can help to regenerate the immune system. It achieves this by triggering the production of new white cells that fight off infections keeping you free from infections and diseases.

Fasting allows your body to eliminate inefficient, worn out, and damaged cells that constitute your immunity system. Researchers believe that intermittent fasting can assist anyone with low immunity to boost their levels in order to prevent infections and stay healthy.

6. Intermittent fasting helps to extend lifespan

There is a strong correlation between intermittent fasting and longevity. Researchers at the University of Chicago in Illinois have discovered that intermittent fasting can delay the development of disorders that usually lead to death. The research has shown that individuals who practice regular fasting do benefit from healthier and longer life compared to those who don't. When your digestive system and metabolic activity are constantly working, then you set in motion the aging process. Fasting produces the opposite reaction. It results in stress within the cells which promotes cell and tissue repair. These anti-aging properties assist in keeping your organs functioning effectively and efficiently.

7. It is excellent for brain health

Your brain is an extremely important organ of the body. Scientists say that what is good for the body is good for the brain. As you fast, your metabolism rates will improve greatly. Improved metabolism helps to reduce oxidative stress, inflammation, and blood sugar levels. According to a report released in 2015 by the Society for Neuroscientists, the brain gets stimulated in different ways. The study shows that intermittent fasting has major benefits for the brain.

When the brain is stimulated, your memory will be enhanced in various ways. Also, this will enhance recovery after an injury while promoting the growth of neurons. Fasting promotes conditions of the brain so that risks of brain conditions such as Parkinson's and Alzheimer's. The research scientists behind this study also claim the fasting improves quality of life as well as cognitive functions of patients with these brain problems.

8. It helps to combat oxidative stress

Oxidative stress is a type of stress that is usually caused by unstable molecules in the body. These unstable molecules are also known as free radicals. These can be extremely dangerous to the body. They cause serious damage to organs and enhance the aging process. They are also thought to play a huge role in the development and onset of cancer and other health conditions.

Intermittent fasting provides an excellent solution to these problems and challenges. Research findings show that regular fasting provides a solution to the challenges posed by free radicals. Basically, as you fast, you activate your stress defenses. These defenses are activated in the body even in the absence of the stressor. As the body begins to break down fats as you fast, it begins to eliminate waste and toxins present in your body. Once cells are cleaned, the rejuvenation process of these cells begins. Fasting will also promote or help to battle inflammation.

9. Intermittent fasting is beneficial to your heart

According to statistics, heart disease is the world's top killer. Millions of Americans will expect to fall victims to heart disease. Some of the risk factors associated with a healthy heart include blood pressure, LDL cholesterol, and others.

Research scientists are of the opinion that regular checkups are essential and it also helps you lose weight. Fasting helps to eliminate bad cholesterol. All these are factors that need to be considered as high-risk indicators of heart disease. When you fast and work out regularly, then these will help lower your risk levels. Reduced bodyweight helps you to be flexible and move fast.

With lower body fat and weight, you are able to move faster and the risk of heart disease will be greatly reduced. It is widely believed that any person who pursues this kind of lifestyle like you and others do will have a healthier heart.

Doctors have known for a long time that individuals who follow a restricted calorie intake once or twice a week will most certainly have better heart health compared to those who do not.

Health Benefits of Calorie Restrictions

There are numerous credible studies that confirm the benefits of calorie restrictions on human health. According to the findings of some of these studies, not only do you benefit from calorie restrictions but that this is an essential requirement if you are to live a long healthy life.

Research done on mice at the John Hopkins University clearly indicates that life-long calorie restriction significantly alters the general structure of gut bacteria or microbiota. This alteration happens in a manner that tends to promote longevity. Therefore, calorie restriction promotes longevity by altering the structure of gut microbiota.

Longevity due to calorie restrictions is more a factor of a reduction in disease states within the body that would otherwise destroy life. There are certain health improvements that are also associated with calorie restrictions. They include improved insulin sensitivity, lower visceral fat levels, lower blood pressure, and reduced inflammation levels.

Intermittent fasting shares similar benefits to calorie restrictions even when you do not strictly restrict daily calorie intake. A review was conducted by research scientists in 2013 at the University of Chicago. This review revealed a wide range of therapeutic benefits that were as a result of intermittent fasting. These benefits are actually possible even when there was no significant reduction in the total amount of calories consumed. In reality, if you choose a specific intermittent fasting protocol, you will still be able to consume the same amount of calories each day like before and still enjoy the benefits of intermittent fasting.

Intermittent Fasting Helps with the Following

- o It reduces inflammation
- o Lowers blood pressure
- o Reduces levels of dangerous visceral fats

- Causes stem cells to start the self-renewal process
- Protects the body against cardiovascular diseases
- Improves the functions of the pancreas
- Activates reduction in oxidative stress and cellular damage
- Prevents or slows down the progression of type II diabetes
- Significantly reduces body weight for overweight and obese persons
- Improves your metabolic efficiency

Advice and Tips for Successful Intermittent Fasting

Drink green tea during fasting. While not essential, it makes the experience easier. Green tea suppresses appetite and curbs hunger pangs.

It is important to drink water when you fast as it will fill your stomach. This sends a message to the brain that you are full and you will feel less hungry.

Be on the lookout for body cues. For instance, if you feel upset or stressed out during your fast, then try and relax. Take some deep breaths and focus closely because this is exactly what hunger does to you.

Stock your house with plenty of healthy foods and snacks. These can include grains, veggies, and lean proteins. If you do this, then you will always feed your body the healthy stuff instead of binging on the wrong food types.

Chapter 6: Food Guide

Intermittent Fasting is a lifestyle that involves a pattern of fasting and eating. It is, therefore, more than just a diet. This lifestyle does not dictate what you should eat but rather when you should have your meals. Even then, if you wish to benefit from this lifestyle, then you really should focus on what you eat.

Changing what you eat is crucial because you will be able to lose weight and gain lean muscle without necessarily having to drastically cut back on your calorie intake. Some dieters prefer having large meals within a shorter period of time. This is, in fact, an excellent way of losing weight while maintaining your muscle mass.

Food and Nutrition

Nutrition is simply the science about the nutrients found in foods and the relationship between these nutrients and growth, reproduction, good health, and disease.

According to Lauren Harris-Pincus, MS, RDN, who is also the author of "The Protein-Packed Breakfast Club", if you want to enjoy all the benefits of intermittent fasting then you should resort to clean eating. This means eating fresh foods, natural produce, whole grains, and lean meats as often as possible.

Nutrient-Dense Foods

Experts agree that having a well-balanced diet is essential for weight loss and maintaining energy levels. It is also crucial if you are to stick with this lifestyle. Therefore, if you want to be healthy, lose weight, and enjoy all other benefits of intermittent fasting, then you should focus on eating nutrient-dense foods.

These include seeds, beans, nuts, veggies, fruits, whole grains as well as lean proteins and dairy products.

Your target really should be foods that improve health such as unprocessed foods, those rich in fiber, whole foods, and foods that offer flavor and variety. Therefore, ensure that you eat from a wide range of foods. Here is a list of some of these foods.

Water: While you may not be eating for most of the day, you should still hydrate your body. All the organs in your body really need water in order to function optimally. While the amount of water than people drink varies, you should aim at having urine that is a pale yellow color at all times. Should the color be dark yellow then it means that you are dehydrated.

If you do get dehydrated, then you are likely to suffer from fatigue, headaches, and dizziness. This is even worse when you are fasting so always ensure that you stay hydrated at all times. Should you not like the taste of water, then you can add a slice of lemon or cucumber or perhaps a few mint leaves.

Cruciferous vegetables: One of the crucial ingredients for your diet is fiber. This is found in plenty in cruciferous vegetables like cauliflower, Brussels sprouts, and broccoli. Fiber is essential for eliminating waste, preventing constipation, and keeping your digestive system in excellent working condition. Fiber also makes you feel full so you do not need to snack throughout the day.

Fish: You should aim to eat at least 8 ounces of fish each week or more if possible. There are great reasons why this is important. Fish is not just delicious but is excellent for your health. This is because it contains a number of excellent nutrients such as vitamin D, vitamin E, proteins, and other healthy oils like omega-3 fatty acids. If you will be fasting most of the day, then you will be better off with a food that provides maximum nutrition. Fish is also considered a "brain food" as it provides the brain with essential nutrients required for optimum performance.

Avocado: One reason that avocados are so popular is because they contain plenty of good fats. While some may wonder why choose a fruit with so many calories when weight loss is the goal, this is a very satiating food. Also, the oils contained in avocado fruit are monounsaturated. This means that they are great for the body. Avocado will keep you feeling full most of the day so you can go about your business even if you are fasting.

Berries: If you love smoothies, then you probably top them up with fruit. One of the most nutritious yet delicious fruits out there is the berry. You have a wide range of berries to choose from. They range from strawberries to blueberries and all others. They all happen to be a great source of vitamin C. Just one cup delivers more than your daily recommended allowance. There is also a recent study that found that individuals who consumed a diet rich in bio-flavanoids have very little chance of gaining weight in the immediate and long-term future. Both strawberries and blueberries are rich in bio-flavanoids among other nutrients.

Legumes and beans: Some of the foods best for the provision of energy include beans and legumes. While you should go slow on carbs, it doesn't hurt to have some low-calorie carbs on your menu. Think about foods such as lentils, peas, black beans, and chickpeas. Beans and legumes are definitely low-carb foods that you should have regularly. These are all known to aid with weight loss even when you simply eat normally with no calorie restrictions.

Potatoes: People tend to believe that all white foods are bad for you. However, some white foods such as potatoes are really great for you. Studies have shown that potatoes are very satiating. Other studies point to the fact that potatoes can actually aid with weight loss. However, if you are to benefit from potatoes then they should constitute a part of a healthy diet. You can eat them boiled, grilled, and as part of a stew. Try and avoid potato chips and French fries versions as these do not support weight loss and are not good for you.

Whole grains: People still find it hard to believe that you can lead a healthy lifestyle and still eat carbs. The two seem to be from totally different worlds. However, whole grains are actually excellent for your body. They are packed full of proteins and fiber. Therefore, eating just a small amount of whole grains will go a long way in getting you to feel satiated.

Studies also indicate that your metabolism is spiked up when you choose to eat whole grains instead of refined grains. You should, therefore, include whole grains as part of your regular diet. Make sure you get out of your comfort zone and try out all sorts of grains include Kamut, millet, bulgur, faro, sorghum, amaranth, spelt, and so much of what is out there. You will be surprised that whole grains actually boost your metabolism.

Nuts: Nuts are pretty high in calories compared to numerous other snacks. However, they contain oils that are great for the body. Good fat is what they contain and this is the difference between nuts and other snacks, most of which contain dangerous fats. In fact, research does suggest that the polyunsaturated fats in walnuts can change completely change certain markers in the body to make you feel full instead of hungry.

You should generally not worry about putting on weight due to the healthy oils in nuts. Nuts such as walnuts have much lower calories than indicated on the label. These nuts also do not get fully digested and some parts remain intact and non-absorbed.

Eggs: Eggs are an excellent source of protein and very nutritious. A single large contains about 6 grams of protein and can be prepared in a matter of minutes. You need to stay satiated and build muscle during the day. There is a study (https://www.ncbi.nlm.nih.gov/pubmed/20226994) which found that men who consumed an egg for breakfast rather than junk food ate less throughout the day and also felt less hungry in comparison. Therefore, next time you want to eat some awesome and filling proteins, try and remember to boil an egg.

Include Probiotics in Your Diet

Probiotics are essential and should be included as part of your diet. They enhance the performance of the gut as well as the rest of the digestive system. The tummy loves it when you provide it with diversity and consistency.

This means that whenever you are hungry, the microbiota gut bacteria are not happy. When there are problems with the digestive system, then you will suffer from constipation and other troubles. Constipation gives you sleepless nights and terrible conditions like constipation. Fortunately, there are plenty of options out there when it comes to micro-bacteria or probiotics. If you sense problems with your digestive system, you can add foods rich in probiotics such as kombucha, kefir, and kraut.

Foods to Avoid

There are certain foods that you need to avoid completely. While intermittent fasting does not dictate what foods you should have, there are food groups or types that you should avoid.

1. Deep fried foods: Deep fried foods usually lose all their nutrients. The super-hot frying oils alter the nature of foods so that they are no longer of great value to the body.

2. Simple carbs and simple sugars: These are often digested very fast and will cause you to feel hungry very soon thereafter. They will also spike your sugar and leave you craving for more.

3. Processed and packaged foods: These foods are often very low in nutrients and are never fresh. They usually contain large amounts of added sugars, plenty of salt, stabilizers, coloring, and other undesirable additives. These are definitely not good for you. If you have to have processed foods, only have it sparingly once or twice each week.

Best Foods to Eat on Intermittent Fasting

- Ensure that you include a serving of protein with each snack or meal. Examples of suitable proteins include grass-fed beef, chicken breast, whole eggs, Greek yogurt, chickpeas, whey protein, fish, cottage cheese, nutritional yeast, tuna, and beans.

- You should have lots of cruciferous, green, leafy vegetables. these vegetables are packed with lots of minerals, vitamins, micronutrients, flavonoids, and others. They include cabbage, broccoli, spinach, cauliflower, lettuce, and cauliflower

- If you feel like having a sweet snack, then opt for a fruit such as an orange than artificial sweets, candy and so on

- Make sure that your diet includes healthy fats like olive oil, coconut oil, nut butters, nuts, grass-fed butter and so on

- Complex carbs are excellent for your diet. These include brown rice, oats, sweet potatoes, and quinoa. These are excellent foods for weight loss

- You should drink plenty of water throughout the day. Apart from water, you can also take green tea and coffee as you fast

Tips about Food, Meals, and Nutrition

Intermittent fasting is a lifestyle that demands you to limit your food intake. First of all, you will need to get used to eating less than 3 meals per day on fast days. Researchers at the Longevity Institute of the University of Southern California have for the last couple of years studied meal timings, calorie restrictions, and calorie intake. According to their findings, even eating three meals per day could be too much. Basically, you will be healthier if you consume fewer meals each day. Here are some other crucial points from the experts.

Eat breakfast or dinner, but not both: Skipping breakfast every now and then is a great idea to introduce to your life. There are those who are completely used to breakfast and can't do without it. If that is you, then have breakfast and lunch but then skip dinner.

Fill your plate with low-calorie vegetables: low-calorie vegetables are great for you. Not only are they tasty but also fill you up and also do your body plenty of good. Also, choose high protein meals if you can. These fill you up and keep you satiated for the longest time.

Keep your carb intake to a minimum: Carbohydrates are pretty high in calories yet they do not leave you feeling satiated. As such, you are likely to feel hungry again pretty soon. Choose complex carbs which release energy slowly rather than simple carbs. Examples of carbs include sweet potatoes, rice, pasta, Irish potatoes, breakfast cereals, and oats and so on.

Don't shy away from fat: It is a fact that fats are very high in calories and are known to cause obesity. However, while fats are high in calories, they also help to make you feel full. Try and include small amounts of fats with your diet especially when you fast. The focus should be to ensure that your meals are low in carbs and sugars yet high in vegetables and proteins.

Intermittent Fasting and Alcohol

When it comes to alcohol, it is crucial that you do not touch alcohol while fasting. You should first conclude your fasting then eat and ensure that your tummy is full before touching any alcohol. Also, ensure that you drink sufficient amounts of water because alcohol can be very dehydrating. When you hydrate, you avoid dehydration, poor athletic performance, a dry mouth, headaches, and difficulty focusing.

If you have to drink alcohol, do it during your eating window. Drinking on an empty stomach will make you drink a lot faster.

Alcohol is easily absorbed in the stomach. It is absorbed directly into the bloodstream. If you have food in your tummy it will slow down the alcohol uptake. Have a balanced meal if you are going to drink alcohol. Have this meal with your beverage to avoid getting overly intoxicated.

Chapter 7: Getting Started with Intermittent Fasting

When you start this lifestyle change, you will need to adjust your eating habits. Intermittent fasting requires you to deny yourself food for certain times during the day. You need to keep in mind that this is a lifestyle which you will now adopt and follow. Here are some tips to help you get started.

1. Choose your preferred intermittent fasting protocol

There are a number of different protocols out there. They are designed to suit different dieters based on their lives. For example, if you love waking up early and working out in the morning, then you can find a fasting protocol that is best aligned with you. There are those who love working out in the evening while others during mid-morning or early afternoon.

We lead such busy lives today that we hardly have time to stop and eat. If you wish, you can fast for one or two days per week and then not worry about fasting for the rest of the week. You can, as an example, opt to fast on Monday's and Thursday's and then eat normally the rest of the week.

2. Adjust your eating habits

Another serious consideration you will need to make is adjusting your eating habits. While this lifestyle does not dictate the kind of foods you should eat, you should learn how to adjust your diet so that you eat mostly healthy, fresh, and nutritious foods. You also need to watch your calorie intake and avoid processed foods, junk foods, and all other unhealthy options.

Unhealthy eating can lead to undesirable effects such as high blood sugar levels, unregulated hormones, low energy levels, mood swings and so on. If you choose unhealthy food options, then your body will be forced to work extra hard in order to eliminate toxins.

3. Begin the Transition

You should now begin the transition. This is the transition into a lifestyle of fasting on a regular basis. Since you already have a preferred protocol, you should now begin to ease into this protocol. Easing into this protocol could be as simple as delaying your first meal of the day by a few hours and cutting back on late night eating.

You should keep in mind that intermittent fasting is a lot more about the mind than it is about diet and lifestyle. It is crucial at this stage that you adjust your chosen lifestyle. It is similar to the way muscles are trained by starting off with light weights and fewer repetitions. The weights and repetitions are then increased gradually.

Once you begin, proceed slowly but surely. The start process will involve regular adjustments of your diet, eating habits, and fasting hours. Keep improving until you get to a level that you are comfortable with.

4. Find a support group or person

Once you begin the intermittent fasting journey, consider finding people who share your ideals and chosen lifestyle. If you wish to be successful, then you should think about partnering with others who are on a similar lifestyle. There are plenty of places to find such support groups. Think about popular social networking sites like Facebook and Twitter.

5. Consider use of delayed gratification

One approach that works superbly is the delayed gratification process. Think about a child who asks the mother for permission to go out and play with other kids. Instead of a direct yes, the mother may delay approval until a later time. Basically, the delay can be used as a tool to help manage hunger and intermittent fasting. Delay eases the pain of desire.

Reorganize your meals

It is advisable to reorganize your meals so that you eat mostly complex carbohydrates and proteins first. Some of the foods that you need to include in your diet should be fish, lean meats, fruits, vegetables, grains, and others.

You should ensure that you plan your meals on time. When you think about what you will eat later, focus on quality foods such as lean protein, white meats, and complex carbs. These will keep you full for longer and are good for your digestive system. The order of your meals should be complex carbs, then simple carbs, and eventually any delayed gratification foods you may want.

The One Week Kick-Start Plan for Fat loss and Muscle Growth

One of the ways of starting the intermittent fasting lifestyle plan is by following this one-week plan. There are numerous ways of doing intermittent fasting. Instead of limiting calorie intake, this lifestyle affords you a brief eating window within which you eat all your meals. Therefore, intermittent fasting is not a diet per se, but a healthy lifestyle and way of eating.

One of the most common ways of following this lifestyle is via the 16/8 fasting protocol. This protocol demands that you fast for 16 hours and then have all your meals inside the 8-hour eating window. Plenty of people prefer this protocol because it is much easier to follow. keep in mind that at least 8 hours of this diet include your sleeping time. Therefore, you fast for 8 hours and sleep for an additional 8 hours. Here is a look at the best ways to start this program. While it may sound a little difficult at first, it really is simple once you get used to it. all you need to do is be patient for a while and you will enjoy this lifestyle complete with the body that you will end up in.

71

Monday meal program

- First meal: Chia seeds pudding
- Snack: Orange fruit
- Second meal: Fried chicken salad
- Snack: Muesli bar
- Supper: Chicken curry

Tuesday meal program

- First meal: Whey protein shake
- Snack: Assorted nuts
- Second meal: Vegetarian chickpea salad
- Snack: An apple
- Supper: Quinoa salad

Wednesday meal program

- First meal: A vanilla whey protein shake
- Snack: A protein bar
- Second meal: Tuna salad sandwiches
- Snack: Yoghurt
- Supper: Fried rice with mixed veggies

Thursday meal program

- First meal: Fried eggs
- Snack: Banana
- Second meal: Broccoli and carrot salad
- Snack: Almonds and dark chocolate
- Dinner: Chicken garlic

Friday meal plan

- First meal: coconut chocolate protein balls
- Snack: Scrambled egg
- Second meal: Taco salad
- Snack: Almond nuts

  o Supper: Chicken salad

Saturday meal plan

  o First meal: Paleo breakfast bar
  o Snack: Hummus carrots
  o Second meal: Chickpea and avocado salad
  o Snack: Zucchini chips
  o Dinner: Chicken and fresh vegetables

Sunday meal plan

  o First meal: A protein smoothie
  o Snack: Mixed nuts
  o Second meal: Chicken salad
  o Snack: Whey protein
  o Supper: Quinoa salad

Actions for Insane and Rapid Fat Loss

1. Fast for longer: If you want to lose weight very rapidly, then there are a couple of things that you should do. One is to fast regularly. For instance, if you are on the 16-8 fasting protocol, you will fast for 16 hours with an 8-hour eating window. Basically, if you fast for longer, then you will shed more pounds.

Increase your fast days: You can increase the frequency of your fasts. For example, the 5-2 protocol requires you to eat normally for five days and then fast for 2 days. Instead of fasting for 2 days, consider increasing this to 3 days. This means that for 3 days a week, you will limit your food intake to a maximum of 500 to 600 calories.

2. Consider doing fasted cardio: One of the best ways of losing body fat is through fasted cardio. This is when you do your cardio workouts as you fast. When you work out on an empty stomach, your body will be forced to tap into fat reserves in the body in order to produce energy. Your body will derive the energy it needs to power your workouts from stored fat reserves.

Therefore, if you want to lose weight rapidly, reduce your caloric intake and work out on an empty stomach in order to burn stored fats. However, approach these tactics with caution because you could feel weak, dizzy, or faint.

Chapter 8: Maintaining the Fast

It is crucial that intermittent fasting is maintained for the long term. This is the best way for you to benefit from this amazing lifestyle. Maintaining this lifestyle in the long run, requires focus, dedication, and making the right choices. For instance, you need to make sure that you tailor intermittent fasting so that it works for you.

Make Intermittent Fasting Work for You

There is no single way of making intermittent fasting perfect for everyone. People are different with varying lifestyles and preferences. However, any healthy person can benefit from this lifestyle. This is because it is safe for you and you can practice it as often as you like.

The crucial aspect is to ensure that you are receiving all the nutrition that your body requires. You can choose a particular diet to follow such as the Mediterranean diet or ketogenic diet so as to benefit for the long term.

Try and make intermittent fasting work for you. For instance, if you have to wake up early, need to work the night shift, have a family or spouse and anything of that nature, that your life will still proceed normally even as you adapt the fasting lifestyle. You should also keep trying and experimenting until you find what works for you.

Lastly, you should keep your focus on what you wish to achieve with intermittent fasting. Weight loss is, of course, one of the major benefits but there are numerous other benefits too. They include low blood sugar, lower blood pressure, reduced inflammation, better coronary heart health, and so much more. Focusing on these numerous benefits should motivate you sufficiently to stick with this lifestyle.

Why You Should Stick with Intermittent Fasting Long-Term

1. Effortless fat burning

If you want to lose weight and keep it off in the long run, then your best bet is intermittent fasting. This lifestyle that involves cycles of fasting and eating has been proven over and over again as the best and safest approach to shedding fat, losing weight and keeping it off for the long term.

All other typical diets provide unimpressive results replete with weight regain over time. This can lead to frustrations. Only intermittent fasting lifestyle is able to aid with fat burning that can lead to greater weight loss compared to a typical calorie-restriction diet.

2. End Insatiable Hunger

There is often concern raised about hunger throughout the day as dieters fast. Such concerns are not unfounded based on past experiences with other diets. As you fast, your body will enter the fat-burning mode. However, hunger pangs will fade as soon as fatty acids enter your bloodstream. The brain will not place demands on the body for energy if it starts receiving energy from fat-based fuels. As such, you can expect to feel satiated as you fast.

3. Sufficient energy for your Entire Day

Even as you fast, you are unlikely to feel hungry or lack energy. The reason for this lack of lethargy is that the body will not be relying on fluctuating carbs stores as a source of energy. Carbs are our regular source of energy but can be unreliable when compared to the fast diet. As we fast, the body gets to receive consistent energy so that the body is fueled and not depleted of energy.

4. Intermittent fasting motivates you to make healthy choices

There is sufficient evidence that most dieters who follow intermittent fasting lifestyle tend to stick with it. While this may surprise some, it really is to be expected simply because the benefits are immense. There is a school of thought out there that says our daily willpower is largely limited. This is why people usually give up on ordinary diets that are so restrictive. Intermittent fasting, on the other hand, gives you plenty of leeways to make independent decisions leaving you with an abundant willpower to stick with the lifestyle.

5. Increased longevity

Both calorie restriction and intermittent fasting lifestyles have been proven to slow down or stop the onset of disease and boost health span. If you do not have any chronic conditions such as cancer, heart disease, high blood pressure, or diabetes, then your chances of suffering from these conditions are drastically reduced. These are huge benefits of intermittent fasting yet you do not need to suffer calorie restrictions or limited food choice.

How to Handle Initial Fasting Challenges

Have the right mindset: You really need to have the right mindset when you start fasting. If you start to feel hungry just hours into your fast, then you should try and focus on other more crucial matters. You should make sure that you take precautionary measures such as drinking lots of water, drinking coffee or green tea. These will keep your hunger at bay and allow you to continue with your fast. Always keep in mind the reasons why you adopted this lifestyle and the benefits it affords your entire system.

Learn to discern between psychological and physical hunger: There is a huge difference between physical and psychological hunger. Physical hunger is easily satisfied by eating a meal or even snacking. This type of hunger is felt gradually and is satiated easily without any guilt feelings. Emotional hunger is rather different. This type of hunger can happen suddenly and may feel urgent. It causes specific cravings and causes you to eat a lot more than you should. When you eat due to psychological hunger, you will feel uncomfortably full and you will feel terribly guilty for your actions.

Keep your mind and body active: It is important that you keep as busy as you fast. Keeping busy and focusing on work or other tasks will keep your mind from hunger and food. If you can then you should try and stay occupied. For instance, you should try to immerse yourself in activities that you relish especially during morning hours. You are more productive in the morning so try and stay busy during this period. Keep in mind that even as you fast, you are losing weight and shedding off the unhealthy fats.

Take a tablespoon or two of Psyllium Husk: This is an edible soluble fiber that does your body plenty of good. Psyllium Husk is also a prebiotic and is a common dietary supplement. If you take this product on a regular basis, it will expand and draw water from the colon. It is an efficient colon cleanser and will eliminate waste efficiently. Even as it works on your body, you will not feel any abdominal discomfort such as bloating. Also, Psyllium will promote a healthy heart and positively impact cholesterol levels.

Overcoming hunger pangs: Dieters generally suffer from hunger pangs only for a brief period of time. Most people claim that hunger pangs tend to disappear within a period of two to three weeks. Hunger is barely noticeable beyond the fourth week.

How to Make Intermittent Fasting Easy on the Body

1. Take Water and Beverages to Stay Hydrated

This is one of the simplest tips yet it is mostly avoided by dieters. It is advisable to drink plenty of water throughout the day and remain hydrated. You should also drink other non-caloric beverages. These will not only hydrate you but will help to stave off hunger. Sometimes water may taste a little bland. In such a case, you may add a dash of lemonade. You should not worry about making numerous trips to the bathroom. Water flushes out toxins from the body and keeps you hydrated.

2. Drink Bone Broth

Sometimes you may wish to increase your energy levels by taking bone broth. Bone broth contains almost zero calories yet it helps to keep hunger pangs at bay. Research shows that bone broth actually suppresses appetite. It also has anti-obesity properties and does a great job at regulating blood sugar. Take bone broth whenever hunger pangs bother you persistently.

3. Consult a nutrition expert

If you want, you may consult a nutritionist and get insights on how to manage the fast. This health expert can expertly guide you and advise you on the changes that you are embarking on. Whenever that you are unsure of something, you should reach out and ask for assistance or advice.

Tracking Progress and Keeping Motivated

A lot of people start a dieting protocol but then give up shortly thereafter. The reason for this is often because of lack of motivation, little or no progress, and a tough regime or rules and restrictions. Fortunately, this is hardly the case when it comes to intermittent fasting. First, you should accept that intermittent fasting is a lifestyle and not an overnight fast. Losing weight takes a bit of time. Therefore be a little more patient in order to see success eventually.

1. Use a mirror to observe your progress

As soon as you begin this lifestyle, take a look at yourself in the mirror. Observe your body closely and identify the sections that require some work and those where layers of fat need to be worked on. If possible, take photos of yourself then keep observing and noting any changes that occur over time.

2. Eat a variety of foods

Rather than consume one type of food or a small variety, you should consider eating a wider variety of foods. Eating just one food type or a limited variety eventually becomes boring. It is ideal to find out more about the foods that you should eat. These should be unprocessed, healthy, fresh, and whole. Once you discover a variety of foods, you will then be able to enjoy your meals even more.

3. Find a suitable partner

You may not know it but working with a partner is highly recommended. This partner could be a spouse, a sibling, or a close friend who shares your passions. You can go through the entire diet and meal plans with this partner and then be each other's coach during workouts. A partner is great to have because you can motivate each other, go shopping together, and generally share this journey with someone close to you.

4. Use before and after photos

Photos are crucial because they motivate you. It is often encouraging when you view photos and note how far you have come. Photos are very motivational. Think about the before – after photos in 3, 6, and 9 months. The difference is amazing and the results will definitely impress you and encourage many others.

5. Other things you can do

There are a couple of other things that you can do to keep track of progress, observe changes and developments, and stay motivated. Grab some weighing scales and weigh yourself. If you can determine your weight, you should then weight yourself occasionally, probably once every two weeks. Note down measurements each time you measure your weight.

You can also take measurements around your waist, chest, arms, and legs. If you lead a suitable intermittent fasting, then you will notice a reduction in these measurements. For instance, your waist measurements should reduce drastically when you fast. You should also work out regularly. Regular workouts and physical activity help to keep you physically fit and assist with weight loss.

You should also check any skin folds that you have. Skin folds constitute excessive skin which becomes visible due to fat loss around the body. If you follow these simple tips and ideas, then there is no doubt that you will attain your weight loss goals.

Chapter 9: Diseases Treated or Cured

Fasting has been part of the human culture for centuries. Doctors have advocated the use of fasting for different reasons including treatment and diagnosis of disease. In recent years, intermittent fasting has emerged as a reliable pathway for treating numerous conditions and diseases. There is anecdotal evidence as well as numerous testimonies from individuals who have experienced healing of one disease or another. Some patients have provided credible evidence of chronic conditions getting cured.

1. Type II Diabetes

Can intermittent fasting cure type II diabetes? This is very possible. The reason is that intermittent fasting can help to lower your blood sugar levels. These levels can be so low, such that you may not require the use of medication.

This idea of using intermittent fasting to treat diabetes has actually been fronted by a medical doctor and kidney specialist, Dr. Jason Fung. Dr. Fung works as a nephrologist at the Intensive Dietary Management Clinic in Toronto, Canada. In the course of his work, he came across numerous patients suffering from diabetes and kidney failure.

He has been using intermittent fasting to help treat diabetes in his patients with excellent outcomes. Apparently, type II diabetes is the most common form of diabetes and accounts to 80% - 90% of cases. It is associated with obesity, unhealthy eating, and usually manifests later in life.

A major aspect of diabetes is insulin resistance. The body usually produces the hormone insulin in order to regulate blood sugar. Insulin facilitates the transfer of glucose in the blood into the cells for use as energy. However, for some unexplained reasons, body tissues are sometimes unresponsive to insulin such that there is too much glucose in the blood.

Patients are normally put on medication that helps to direct glucose into the cells. However, according to Dr. Fung, this is the wrong approach. Intermittent fasting can help to regulate blood sugar and effectively help to treat type II diabetes. When you fast, the body is able to burn off the excess sugar which causes the cells and tissues to become responsive to insulin once more.

Type II diabetes is an entire reversible condition according to Dr. Fung. By fasting regularly, patients tend to lose weight and insulin resistance is overcome. In many instances, patients even stop taking medication.

2. Alzheimer's and Parkinson's Diseases

We have already heard about the power of intermittent fasting and how to can cleanse the body and improve health. However, it has been established that intermittent fasting is able to positively affect certain neurodegenerative diseases like Parkinson's and Alzheimer's.

There is concrete evidence, according to a study by Dr. Mark Mattson of the John Hopkins School of Medicine. The study reveals that intermittent fasting causes the brain to perform in much healthier ways. According to his research findings, fasting a couple of times each week enhances neural connections in a part of the brain known as the hippocampus.

How this helps with neurodegenerative diseases

According to research findings, Dr. Mattson believes that fasting challenges the brain. In response, the brain activates certain stress responses known as adaptive stress responses. These help the brain to cope with the disease. When viewed from an evolutionary perspective, it makes good sense why the brain should be responding so well even when you have had any nourishment for hours.

Fasting turns fat into ketones to produce energy. The process encourages a healthy transformation in the region of the brain that is crucial for memory and learning and overall brain health. This actually works and scientists are excited. Burning fat to produce ketones helps the brain to transform in response to stress. The same thing occurs when we exercise. Dr. Mattson advises patients to attempt two different of performing intermittent fasting. These are the 5:2 protocol and the time-restricted protocol. Dr. Matt also advises some regular physical activity. Exercising is a requirement for this fasting-inspired healing approach.

3. Multiple Sclerosis

In patients suffering from multiple sclerosis, their immune system will wrongfully attack links that attach nerve cells together and prevents them from properly communicating. The immune system not only attacks the nerve links but also causes them harm. This results in undesirable outcomes such as chronic pain, muscle weakness, coordination problems, and fatigue.

Unfortunately, there is currently no cure for multiple sclerosis victims. Current treatment options available to patients only help to manage symptoms. There have been suggestions that dietary interventions could help the body battle this condition.

Researchers from the Washington University School of Medicine in St Louis, MO, believe that interventions such as following the intermittent fasting protocol can help in the management of this condition. One of the research scientists involved in this study, Dr. Laura Piccio says that there is anecdotal evidence about patients who have regained the ability to walk after starting the intermittent fasting lifestyle. However, the doctor claims that this fasting lifestyle greatly helps with the management of symptoms of multiple sclerosis. This makes a huge difference in the lives of patients who live with this chronic condition.

The researchers first conducted tests in the lab with mice models and obtained impressive results. They then tried intermittent fasting on human beings and the outcomes were absolutely phenomenal. The results of the study have been published in the Cell Metabolism journal.

4. High Blood Pressure

Fasting has huge benefits for your heart health and consequently high blood pressure. According to cardiologist Dr. Ahmed, MD, fasting for short periods of time on a regular basis has numerous advantages to the body and generally to your health. It basically pays to limit your calorie intake.

When you fast, you generally lose weight. Weight loss leads to less work for the heart. Fasting also stresses the body sufficiently in a positive manner. The heart becomes stronger and no longer struggles to pump blood.

Research on health benefits of intermittent fasting was published in Nutrition and Healthy Aging journal in June 2018. The findings of the research show that intermittent fasting helps you lose weight and lowers blood pressure. The study focused on obese individuals and they all lost substantial amounts of weight. Plenty of other crucial markers also indicated remarkable improvements.

These include cholesterol, insulin resistance, and fat mass. They all decreased remarkably which in return support the reduction in high blood pressure. The researchers support the 16/8 protocol which supports impressive blood pressure reduction.

5. Heart and Cardiovascular Diseases

Some of the major causes of heart and cardio diseases include excessive body weight, high cholesterol levels, diabetes, and high blood pressure. Researchers have shown that intermittent fasting or restricting food and drink can significantly improve risk factors related to the heart and cardiovascular system.

One study shows that individuals who follow the intermittent fasting lifestyle have better heart health than those who do not follow such a lifestyle. If you lose weight because of intermittent fasting and shed off fat, then your coronary health and cardiovascular system will be in much better shape.

Also, intermittent fasting couples with an active lifestyle will lead to lower blood sugar. It also reduces your levels of low-density lipoproteins sometimes referred to as bad cholesterol.

6. Brain Health

Intermittent fasting has been shown to reduce inflammation throughout the body. It is also an excellent weight loss tool and great for supercharging the brain. Most chronic diseases that we face are as a result of inflammation. These include diabetes, dementia, Alzheimer's, and so on.

Intermittent fasting reduces inflammation through autophagy, ketones, and insulin management. Also, when we fast, more brain cells are created. According to Dr. Mark Mattson of John Hopkins University, fasting has been shown to rapidly increase neurogenesis in the brain. The term neurogenesis refers to the creation or development of new brain cells and related nerve tissues. Fasting also boosts the production of a protein known simply as BDNF which is a miraculous growth protein. This protein helps the brain to grow, change, and adapt to new and changing environments.

7. Cancer

Intermittent fasting is mostly used to boost weight loss. However, it is known to have numerous other benefits ranging from brain health to protection against diseases such as diabetes. Patients suffering from different types of cancers will benefit immensely by adopting an intermittent fasting lifestyle.

There is widely accepted evidence that that fasting, especially intermittent fasting slows and hinders the growth of cancerous tumors. Intermittent fasting also reduces treatment side effects, supports chemotherapy treatment making it more effective, prevents recurrences, and drastically increases survival rates of patients.

While there is still a lot of research going on, current verifiable information shows that intermittent fasting helps to fight cancer, reduces chances for any new cancer cells and supports healing including enhancing chemotherapy and other treatment options. Fasting also denies cancer tumors the nutrition they need to grow and thrive.

8. Gut Health

Intermittent fasting is beneficial for your gut. It promotes gut health in different ways. The human gut contains a myriad of microbes that include fungi, viruses, and bacteria of all sizes and shapes. There are over a thousand species of these microbes in your gut and they greatly affect and impact your health.

Gut microbiota can alter the way the body metabolizes food. They even let the brain known when we are hungry and when we are full. It is now evident that fasting has a huge effect on gut microbiota. By fasting and improving the quality of nutrients, we positively affect gut microbiota.

The body has for thousands of years been used to fasting and being calorie free. It is only in recent years that we had access to food on a 24-hour basis, 7 days a week. By cutting back on nutrition, the digestive system takes a break and the gut bacteria take a break. The quality of gut microbial and their nature improves remarkably when we fast. You can find out a lot more information about this by following this link. Food scarcity is really what our bodies had been used to. We thrive when there is a temporary shortage. The stress caused by fasting helps the body to perform at optimum levels.

87

9. Autoimmune Disease

There are research studies that have shown potential benefits of intermittent fasting for autoimmune diseases such as rheumatoid arthritis and fibromyalgia. This lifestyle is also very promising when it comes to other autoimmune diseases like multiple sclerosis, lupus, and so on.

Basically, when you fast for an extended period of time, the body gets an opportunity to relax and rest. Your body takes this opportunity to heal, recover, and repair because it is not busy digesting food or protecting against inflammatory substances in the food we eat.

When it heals, a lot of positive things happen. For instance, it repairs a leaky gut which is the precursor to all autoimmune diseases. A leaky gut is a term that refers to intestinal permeability. When leaks are sealed in the lining of the intestines, the symptoms of autoimmune diseases can then be managed.

10. Obesity and Overweight

Intermittent fasting has been acknowledged by numerous dieters as an effective weight loss tool. In fact, most people who follow this simple lifestyle do so in order to lose weight and keep it off. The reason why intermittent fasting is so popular as a weight loss tool is because it does not involve extreme effort, constant hunger, or calorie counting.

There are a number of studies out that show this to be factual. A test was done where obese individuals structured their meals such that they fasted for a total of 16 hours per day but were allowed to eat anything they wanted in the next 8 hours. The results were impressive and showed how these individuals lost some modest weight.

Now the same group of obese individuals was requested to go without food for 16 hours but then could only eat 350 less calories during the eating window. This study was conducted by Krista Varady, an associate professor of nutrition at the University of Illinois in Chicago. The participants all lost significant amounts of weight. If done correctly and coupled with regular workouts, intermittent fasting will enable overweight and obese persons to lose weight and keep it off.

Chapter 10: Myths, Common Questions, and Considerations for Men and Women

There are numerous benefits that come out of this lifestyle. There are plenty of testimonies as well as anecdotal evidence about people who've lost vast amounts of weight or had a serious condition healed. If you want to enjoy the benefits of intermittent fasting, then you ought to do it correctly. What you need to be able to do is avoid making common mistakes and debunk any myths out there.

Breakfast Myths

For a long time, we grew up believing that breakfast is the most crucial meal of the day. We were advised to never leave the house without having breakfast. However, the question is, is breakfast really the most important meal of the day? Is it advisable to kick-start the day with a full breakfast meal?

Myth 1: Breakfast is crucial and is a healthy option

For a long time, we have believed that breakfast is a crucial morning meal and that you had to have breakfast in order to have a great morning. However, this may not necessarily be true. Not all breakfast meals are equal and some options could be unhealthy. The healthiest breakfast should include a protein, whole grain, 100% fruit juice or a fruit.

Myth 2: Skipping breakfast helps with weight loss

While skipping some meals and cutting back on calories is a great idea, in some instances, it really isn't. Some healthcare experts believe that skipping breakfast can be detrimental to your health in some instances. Hunger may cause you to overindulge later on. You should stick to eating a balanced diet always.

Myth 3: Breakfast is the most crucial meal of the day

We have for a long time believed that breakfast is the most important meal of the day. However, the truth is that there is no single meal that is the most important of the day. The crucial aspect to consider on any meal is the quality and quantity consumed at each meal.

10 Popular Questions on Intermittent Fasting

Question 1: What is intermittent fasting?

Intermittent fasting is an eating pattern where you cycle between the period of eating and fasting. It is not a diet that tells you to eat one type of food and not eat another food type. However, it is a lifestyle where you fast for a couple of hours, usually 16 hours per day and then have your meals in the remaining time period.

Question 2: What are the benefits of this lifestyle?

Intermittent fasting has numerous benefits. Most people follow this lifestyle in order to lose weight and keep it off. With intermittent lifestyle, you lose weight gradually which means you lose it possibly for good and instead strong, lean muscle.

You can expect increased life expectancy. Studies at the National Institute of Ageing show that animals tend to age slower and live longer if they eat fewer calories. You will notice an improvement in your hormone performance. For instance, you can expect reduced insulin levels, an increase in HGH or human growth hormone, and a reduction in blood sugar levels.

These all support weight loss, lower risk of heart disease and diabetes, and for maintaining lean muscle mass. Intermittent fasting promotes a healthy body by eliminating inflammation in the body.

4. Why and how does intermittent fasting burn fat?

When you limit your calorie intake, there is less glucose on the body. This signals the body to rely more on stored fats than from glucose derived from carbs in your diet. Since the body needs energy to function, it will reach into stored fats and start burning them in order to produce the energy it needs.

5. What makes it so effective?

One of the reasons why intermittent fasting is so powerful is mostly due to the adaptive response from cells. The response results in a reduction in inflammation and oxidative stress. The body also improves cellular production and optimizes the body's metabolism. Intermittent fasting helps the body to handle stress much better especially when cells have to cope with nutrition limitations.

6. What types of intermittent fasting protocols are out there?

There are many ways of doing intermittent fasting. There are different protocols that you can follow. We have 5-2 protocol, the 16/8 protocol, and the alternate day fasting protocol. There is also the 24-hour fast that you can do probably twice or more times per month. There is generally no one protocol that is better than the other. It is simply advisable that you identify one that works for you and stick by it.

7. Where do I begin?

Once you determine that you wish to pursue this kind of lifestyle, you should then think and plan how to begin the journey. Plan to begin fasting on a particular day. It could be a Monday or any other day of the week. The night just before you begin is your first night before intermittent fasting. Ensure that you eat a meal loaded with protein, complex carbs, and vegetables. Complex carbs and proteins will keep you feeling full for much longer. When you wake up in the morning, you will already have fasted for eight hours. At this point, you should go about your business as usual. Take coffee, black tea, or even water should you start feeling hungry again.

8. How do I do intermittent fasting for weight loss?

According to experts, the simplest way to lose weight with an intermittent fasting lifestyle is to fast once per week. Ideally, we lose weight when we consume fewer calories than we burn. One-day fast means once you have your evening meal, you will then eat nothing for the rest of the time until the following day's dinner. As you fast, your body will rely on stored fat to generate energy.

9. What foods are best after breaking the fast?

Quality nutrition is crucial if you want to enjoy the benefits of fasting. If you end your fast around dinner time, then you should have your dinner right there and then. However, if you end your fast around four in the afternoon, then you should have a snack as you wait for dinner.

Whatever meal you decide to have, just ensure that it contains sufficient amounts of assorted vegetables, high-quality proteins such as chicken or fish, a carbohydrate like brown rice, sweet potato and so on. Most dieters usually eat clean after a fast. This is highly advisable because healthy eating results in healthy individuals.

10. Can I exercise during my fasting window?

You may sometimes wish to train in a fasted state. This is likely to result in significant weight loss. Fasted training or fasted cardio is quite popular especially with individuals who wish to lose a lot of weight within a short period of time.

On other non-fast days, you can engage in more rigorous workouts. You can go for jogging or even a hill run. Work on your muscle and develop them so that you are both healthy and fit. Always be careful and watch your energy levels before working out.

Specifically Men and Intermittent Fasting – Things to Consider

1. *Stubborn belly fat*: A lot of men carry a pot belly which never seems to go away no matter how hard they work out. Fortunately, intermittent fasting offers you the best solution yet. By following this lifestyle, you are likely to lose the belly fat and have a flat tummy again. Developing abdominal muscles is also possible

2. *Human growth hormone:* As you fast, your body produces higher amounts of HGH. This is an absolutely important hormone that supports growth and development of tissue and muscles. Higher levels of HGH are necessary to keep you looking great and to slow down aging.

3. *Develop strong*, *lean muscle:* Intermittent fasting helps you lose fat and shed pounds. This also presents an excellent opportunity to develop muscles. Anaerobic workouts are crucial if you are to develop a strong body with lean muscles throughout.

You will, therefore, need to work out regularly, eat the right kinds of foods, and fast occasionally.

4. *Improve your fitness level*: As you fast, you should also maintain your fitness levels. It is advisable to work out regularly and live an active lifestyle. If you work out regularly then you will become physically fit and strong. Your challenge will be to maintain this level of fitness for the long term.

5. *Eat smaller portions*: You are probably used to eating fairly large food portions both at home and whenever you eat at a restaurant. These large portions are no good for you. They simply help you to pile up the kilos. Learn to reduce the size of your portions so that you consume only the calories that your body needs.

Specifically Women and Intermittent Fasting – Things to Consider

1. *Weight loss*: You have probably tried just about all diets out there in order to lose weight and keep it off. Fortunately, there is intermittent fasting. This healthy lifestyle will ensure that you lose weight if done correctly. There are ways of speeding up weight loss. These include doing cardio exercises in a fasted state and fasting for longer periods.

2. *Stubborn belly fat*: Just like men women sometimes also struggle with stubborn belly fat. If you work out regularly and reduce your calorie intake, then you will slowly but surely lose fat around your abdomen area and keep it off. Make sure that you follow your preferred fasting protocol as required.

3. *Fasting and hormones*: One of the major differences between males and females when it comes to fasting is how much they are affected by hormones. According to scientists, women's hormones are affected by fasting much more compared to men.

They believe this is because of a protein known as kisspeptin. Fortunately, intermittent fasting can help in the regulation of hormones. When you fast, work out, and eat healthily, your body will better regulate hormones.

4. Hunger cues: Once you begin fasting, you are likely to experience plenty of hunger. A lot of the appetite hormones occur in higher levels in women than in men. Try not to ignore hunger cues. Instead, prepare well for your fasting session by eating well the night before. Increase your protein intake, drink lots of water. Also, fast maybe once or twice a week and on non-consecutive days.

5. Consider crescendo fasting: This is a fasting protocol developed specifically for women. This fasting approach is kinder to the body and will help your hormones to settle down and not bother you that much. There are definite benefits to crescendo fasting. For instance, you can expect to see your energy levels increase, lose both body weight and body fat, and experience almost no hormonal challenges.

Chapter 11: Popular Intermittent Fasting Celebrities

Intermittent fasting lifestyle has definitely caught the attention of people around the world. Celebrities have not been left out. Everybody has heard how awesome this lifestyle is and how impressive the results are. This is why a lot of people, including celebrities, are joining the bandwagon.

There have been many diets that made headlines in the past couple of decades. These include the grapefruit diet, the low-fat diet, and even the Master Cleanse. Sadly, they did not last for long. However, intermittent fasting is different because it is not a diet but more of a lifestyle and way of eating. It involves periods of fasting and eating. Most celebrities have endorsed one or two protocols even though there are more than five common ones. Here are some of the celebrities who have chosen the intermittent fasting lifestyle.

1. Jennifer Lopez

One of the best-known celebrities who practices intermittent fasting is Jennifer Lopez, also known as J. Lo. While she is always glamorous, J. Lo works extremely hard to look the way she does. Part of her lifestyle involves not eating anything for a period of eight hours per day. She also works out regularly and eats healthy. This shows how well she takes care of her body and overall health.

2. Nicole Kidman

This Australian actress is also said to be an avid follower of this lifestyle. Like J. Lo, Nicole Kidman prefers to follow the 8-hour fasting rule. She prefers to fast regularly and when she eventually sits down to eat she opts for veggies and lean protein.

3. Justin Theroux

Justin is not just a popular celebrity but is also conscious about his health. This is why his trainer convinced him to follow the intermittent fasting lifestyle. Since he discovered this lifestyle, Justin has been fasting for 12 hours between 7.00 pm and 7.00 am and eats only outside of these hours.

4. Beyoncé

One of the leading female artists of all time is Beyoncé Carter. Beyoncé, or Bey as she is popularly known, has been following this lifestyle for a couple of years now. While she has never confirmed it, numerous outlets have confirmed that she does. Beyoncé looks great, is superbly fit, and seems not to age. All these can probably be attributed to intermittent fasting.

5. Terry Crews

Terry was among the very first celebrities to come out and proclaim his love for this lifestyle. He also follows it religiously. His first meal each day is at 2.00 pm. His eating window, which is only 8 hours long, stretches to 10.00 pm. He fasts every single day for 16 hours but enjoys a cup of coffee or tea as he fasts. Apart from fasting, he also works out regularly and has developed some serious muscles.

6. Hugh Jackman

We all love Hugh Jackman and his excellent acting skills. He was also among the very first celebrities to come out in support of intermittent fasting. like Terry Crews, he too prefers to fast for 16 hours during his fasting days and then has all his meals in the 8-hour eating window.

7. Antoni Porowski

Even Antoni is an ardent intermittent fasting adherent. While he does not flaunt this lifestyle, he is keen on maintaining his health and fitness. He usually has his first meal at around 12.00 noon and then keeps this eating window open until 8.00 pm in the evening. He then eats nothing until noon the following day. His amazing good looks, lean physique, and easy going nature highlight all the aspects of intermittent fasting.

Other celebrities

There are plenty of other celebrities who follow this fasting lifestyle. They include Liv Tyler, Miranda Kerr, and Ben Affleck. After becoming aware of the numerous benefits of intermittent fasting, they all chose to pursue it.

A lot of these celebrities prefer to follow the fast diet where they fast for 2 days and then eat normally for 5 days. They find this protocol easier to follow and gentle on the body. Many celebrities were made aware of this lifestyle through a TV documentary. They love this particular lifestyle because it actually works and results are very visible. Intermittent fasting has also been tried successfully and proven to work effectively.

Others who have chosen to pursue this lifestyle include Fiona Becket of the Guardian and Kate Middleton's uncle. They are both of the opinion that this lifestyle has made a huge impact on other people's lives and they too would love to enjoy similar benefits.

Conclusion

Intermittent fasting provides one of the most effective lifestyle changes known to man. Those who have turned to this lifestyle have seen such amazing changes and continue to enjoy such a good quality of life. It is why many concede the switch to this lifestyle as the best decision they have ever made in their lives.

This lifestyle is very simple indeed. Unlike other diets and eating fads, it places no demands on its followers other than the requirement to fast for a period of time and then eat during a brief eating window. Such simple requirements have surprisingly great outcomes.

Starting out is really simple. Your first step is to simply understand all about this lifestyle, how it works, and all its benefits. Once you understand and accept the theory aspect, you will then need to start applying it. The transition is absolutely simple. Once you are able to make the transition, you will be able to indulge in this lifestyle and overcome all initial challenges.

It is even easier to follow this lifestyle because there are numerous protocols to choose from. You will not be compelled to follow a particular protocol but will be free to choose the method that you like. The lifestyle is also accommodating and this allows you to make certain changes so that this fasting program suits your lifestyle. And should you make mistakes along the way, you should not despair and give up. Mistakes are part and parcel of the learning process. Simply shake off the dust and start again.

The benefits of intermittent lifestyle are numerous. Intermittent fasting enables you to lose weight and keep it off. It promotes a healthy body by minimizing inflammation. Intermittent fasting helps to cure diseases and treat certain conditions so that you eventually get to enjoy optimum health. If you encounter difficulties, then you should find a reliable individual to consult with. For instance, find a book to read, a website, or an experienced person and talk to them. It is also great if you can find someone to partner with in this journey. Identify a friend, a spouse or close family member and work together. It is always easier when you have someone to encourage and support you along the way.

Motivation: If you need inspiration or motivation, then consider joining a group of individuals who share the same interest. There are plenty of groups across different social media. Find a group, engage members, and share your experiences and challenges. You are bound to find a willing partner, listening ear, and helpful advice. The benefits of this lifestyle are numerous and you should share in these benefits. Remember to drink plenty of water as you fast and exercise on a regular basis. You are bound to succeed if you pursue this lifestyle correctly and adhere to it diligently. Take photos at different stages and note the amazing changes taking place as you follow this amazing lifestyle.

If you enjoyed this book, please leave me a positive review on Amazon as it keeps me being able to produce quality books. Thank you

Modern Ketogenic Diet

Using the High-Fat And Low-Carb Hack Through The Keto Diet To Shred Fat And Feel Healthy Again (Rapid Weight Loss, Meal Plans, Healthier Lifestyle)

Elliot Cutting

Introduction: The Keto Diet

Most people shorten the Ketogenic diet down and call it the "Keto diet." This word was created because while following this diet, your body creates fuel molecules called *Ketones*. Ketones get used as an alternate source of fuel for our bodies and the body uses these when its glucose supply gets low.

If you don't eat many carbs, your body will produce *Ketones*. This holds true if your protein intake is kept at moderate levels. If you eat too much protein, the body could turn it into sugar.

Your liver can create Ketones from the fat that has been stored in your body. The body will then use the Ketones for fuel for several parts of the body including the brain. The sad part is that our brains can't run off fuel we get from fat. It only gets fuel from glucose or *Ketones*.

While doing a Ketogenic diet, your whole body will change its fuel supply and be able to run entirely off of fat. This causes your insulin level to drop and your body to burn more fat. Your body will be accessing the fat that it has stored over the years and begin to burn it. This is a great diet if you are trying to lose weight and on top of that there are other benefits such as better mental awareness, steady energy supply, and less hunger.

Low Carbs

The only way that this diet will work correctly is by eating a very small amount of carbs. The fewer carbs you eat, the better your chances of losing weight. A Keto diet is very strict with low-carbs. You will only be able to eat 20 grams or less of net carbs every day.

Once you have achieved your weight loss goals, you can start to increase the number of carbs you eat. This will need to be done slowly so that you don't end up gaining the weight you lost.

Covering The Basics

It is a must that you follow this diet firmly in order to get better and faster results.

In theory, a Ketogenic diet is simple—low-carbs, high fat. This doesn't exactly tell you what you can and can't eat. There is a complete list of foods you can eat later on in the book, but for now here is a quick overview:

- Meats including organ meat.
- Fish and seafood
- Heavy fats such as bacon fat, tallow, butter, olive oil, coconut oil, ghee, and lard.
- Eggs
- Berries like blueberries, strawberries, and raspberries.
- Nonstarchy vegetables—all the leafy greens you care to eat.

Your typical day could look something like this:

- Breakfast could include bacon and eggs.
- Lunch could include a cup of bone broth with a chicken salad.
- Dinner might consist of a steak, side of veggies, and a dessert that is Keto-friendly.

Some people have to snack between meals. If you are like this, good choices are meat sticks, broth, cheese sticks, celery sticks, and nuts. You have to watch how many snacks you eat since these will make your total calorie count go up.

The Keto diet is very easy to personalize and you have the ability to experiment and figure out what will work best for you due to the various food options. Some people may realize that they need more fats in their diet, and others might be able to eat fewer carbs.

Ketosis

Let's take a closer look at it and figure out what it actually is. Ketosis is a natural state that the body goes into when it is fueled by fat. This will happen when you fast or follow a strict low-carb diet such as the Keto diet.

There are several benefits in allowing your body to get into Ketosis, these being increased health, performance, and weight loss. There are some side effects to consider just like anything else such as if you have type 1 diabetes or other diseases, too much Ketosis could be dangerous.

Once your body gets into Ketosis, it produces *Ketones*. As stated above, these small molecules can be used as fuel for the body. The liver converts fat into *Ketones* and releases them into the bloodstream. The body will then use them like glucose.

How to Get into Ketosis

Our bodies can get into Ketosis in two different ways; fasting or a Ketogenic diet. With either one of these ways, the body has limited sources of glucose, causing the body to switch and use fat for fuel. When the hormone insulin gets low, the body will increase its fat burning properties. This means your body now has access to all of your stored fat and melts it.

Scientifically proven, fasting will create ketosis in the body fast than the Keto diet, however most people decide to do the Keto diet because it can be eaten for an indefinite amount of time and you don't have to worry about hunger pains and food time management.

Fuel for Our Brains

Most people think the brain needs carbs for fuel. The brain actually can't burn carbs when you eat them, but if carbs aren't available, it burns Ketones.

This is needed for basic human survival. Because our bodies can only store carbs for one or two days, the brain will just shut down after several days without food. Alternatively, it would begin converting muscle protein into glucose fast in order to keep working. This is not very effective. This means we will waste away quickly. If this is the way the body actually works, then the human race would not have survived before food became available all day and every day.

The human body has evolved in order to work smarter. Normally, the body will have stored enough fat so that someone could survive a few weeks without eating anything at all. Ketosis a process of survival that happens to make sure our brains can run on fat stores.

Ketosis and Ketoacidosis

There are a lot of misconceptions about Ketosis. The main one is thinking it is the same thing as Ketoacidosis. Ketoacidosis is a rare but dangerous condition that happens to people who have type 1 diabetes. Sometimes even health care professionals mix these two things up. It might be because the names are very similar, and there isn't a lot of knowledge between the differences.

Ketosis is a natural state for the body, and our bodies control it all by itself. Ketoacidosis is a malfunction in the body where it creates an excessive and unregulated amount of Ketones. This could cause symptoms like stomach pain, nausea, and vomiting, which can be followed by confusion and even a coma. This requires urgent medical treatment and could end up being fatal.

So before someone gets this diet confused when you're having a conversation about it, you won't freak out and you will know exactly what they're talking about.

Reaching Optimal Level of Ketosis

This is the point that everybody who does the Ketogenic diet wants to get to. When you have reached the optimal level of Ketosis, your body will begin to burn fat at the best speed. To reach this level of Ketosis, you have to follow a low-carb, high-fat diet, as we stated above. You need to keep your macros at their optimal range. There aren't any specific tricks that will help you do this, just following the steps in this book and experiencing the diet for yourself will leave you with the answers you need.

Here are the different Ketone levels that you might have:

- Less than 0.5 means you haven't reached Ketosis yet.
- A level between 0.5 and 1.5 is a light level of Nutritional Ketosis. You might lose some weight, but you aren't at the optimal level.
- Levels around 1.5 to 3 is considered to be at the optimal level and is best for losing the most weight.
- Levels that are over 3 aren't needed. High levels don't help you at all. It might harm you because it means you aren't eating enough food.

Most people think they have been eating a strict Keto diet but when they measure their blood Ketone levels, they get surprised. Once they measure their levels and they are around 0.2 or 0.5, they realize they aren't near their sweet spot, and they get discouraged.

The trick of getting past this plateau is you have to stick to low-carb sources but also make sure you aren't eating too much protein. Your protein intake doesn't need to be higher than your fat intake. Yes, we have stated that protein doesn't affect your glucose levels as carbs will, but if you consume too many, especially if you eat more protein than fats, this will affect your glucose, effecting your optimal Ketosis.

The trick to working around this is eating more fat. You could easily do this by adding a big dollop of herbed butter to the top of your steak. This may help you not eat as much because fats fill you up quite easily.

Drinking a cup of bulletproof coffee can keep you from getting hungry and eating too much protein. This is simple to do; you just need to add a tablespoon of butter or coconut oil to your coffee every morning.

How to Measure Ketosis

There are many ways you can figure out if you have reached Ketosis. The first way is by measuring Ketones in your blood. This means you will have to buy a meter and prick your finger just like you would to measure blood sugar.

There are many reasonably priced gadgets out there, and it only takes a few seconds to find out what your blood Ketone level is. Most people don't want to go to this extreme just to find out what their Ketone level is, but is the most accurate and effective.

You will need to measure your blood Ketones first thing every morning on a fasted stomach. You can look at the levels we listed earlier to figure out if you are in Ketosis.

These meters measure the amount of BHB that's in your blood. This is the main Ketone that is present in the blood when you are in Ketosis. The biggest problem with this method is having to draw blood.

These kits will cost around $30 to $40 and might cost around $5 for every test. This is the reason most people that decide to test this way, just perform a test each week or so.

We've covered the most expensive way to figure out if you are in Ketosis but there are seven other ways to tell if you are in Ketosis.

1. Bad breath

    This doesn't sound pleasant but people have often stated that they have bad breath when they have reached Ketosis. This is a normal side effect. People have stated that their breath will smell fruitier.

    This is caused by elevated Ketone levels. The big culprit is the Ketone acetone that the body excretes through your breath and urine. You might not like the idea of having bad breath; but it is a great way to know if you are in Ketosis. Most people will brush their teeth more often or chew some sugar-free gum.

2. Weight loss

   This is the best way to tell if you are in Ketosis. When you first start the Keto diet, you will see a quick drop in weight, but this is normally just water weight. When you experience another drop in weight, this will be your fat stores being burnt. This is another way to know you are in Ketosis.

3. Ketones in your breath and urine

   If you don't like having to prick your finger, you can measure blood Ketones by using a breath analyzer. This monitors acetone, which is one of the three Ketones that will be in your book when you reach Ketosis.

   This will let you know when your Ketone levels have hit Ketosis since acetone only leaves the body when you have reached nutritional Ketosis. These breath analyzers are fairly accurate but not as accurate as the blood monitor.

   Another way you could check for Ketosis is checking for Ketones in your urine every day using special indicator strips. This is a cheap and fast method you can use to assess what your Ketones levels are every day. These methods are not very reliable.

4. Appetite suppression

   Most people report their hunger will decrease when following a Keto diet. The reasons behind this are still being studied. It is thought that the reduction in hunger is due to the increase in protein and vegetable consumption, as well as a change in hunger hormones. The Ketones might also affect how your brain reacts to hunger.

5. Better focus and energy

   Some people have reported feeling sick, tired, or having brain fog when they first start the Keto diet. This is called the Keto flu. People that follow this diet for a long time have reported having better energy and increased focus. Your body will need time to adapt to this new diet. Once you hit Ketosis, your brain begins to burn Ketones for energy. This could take a week or two for it to start happening.

6. Short-term fatigue

Once your body starts making the switch to Keto, it might cause weakness and fatigue. This makes it hard for some people to stick with this diet. This side effect is normal, but it is a way to know that you are hitting Ketosis.

This crappy feeling might last for one week or one month before you actually hit full Ketosis. You can reduce this feeling by taking electrolyte supplements.

7. Short-term performance decrease

Just like this point before, the fatigue may cause a decrease in exercise performance. This is caused by the glycogen stores in your muscles being reduced; this gives you the fuel you need to get through high-intensity exercises. After a week or two, your performance levels will return to normal.

Keto Diet Versus the Atkins Diet

These are the two most popular diets that will reduce your intake of carbs drastically, but let's look at how they compare to each other in terms of results, safety, and difficulty.

The Atkins diet and the Ketogenic diet would be tied in a race for the most popular low-carb diets. Both don't just cut back on carbs, like donuts, cupcakes, and cookies, but they also get rid of some veggies, and most fruits. They limit the number of carbs so much that it makes you enter into Ketosis; this makes the body burn fat for fuel once your glucose stores have been depleted. Ketosis plays a huge role in both these diets, and it can also affect how easy it is to stick with them.

Let's go through the Atkins diet quickly. It was introduced in 1972 by Robert Atkins, who was a cardiologist. The original diet, that is now called Atkins 20, had four phases. The first phase had a lot of restrictive rules.

Proteins and fats in the Atkins diet are both fair game but carbs are extremely restricted to around 20 and 25 grams of net carbs. This is the total carbs minus the dietary fiber. All of these carbs need to come from veggies, cheese, seeds, and nuts. This phase will last until you are about 15 pounds away from your goal weight.

Phase two brings your carb amount to about 25 to 50 grams, and you can eat foods like cottage cheese, yogurt, and blueberries. This is going to last until you are ten pounds away from your goal weight.

During phase three, you will up your carb intake to between 50 and 80 grams of net carbs while you try to find the right balance. This means you have to find how many carbs you can eat before your weight loss stalls? This part has to be done slowly and with some trial and error to find how many carbs you can eat without gaining any weight.

When you have found that number, and have maintained it for one month, you will enter phase four. This will be your lifetime maintenance. This part will focus on keeping up with habits that you created during the third phase. You can consume up to 100 grams of net carbs each day as long as you don't begin gaining weight.

There are many different moving parts when talking about the Atkins diet. With the Keto diet, you can only eat one way for the whole diet. You are going to lower your carb intake to about five percent of your daily calorie intake. Because of this, you will enter Ketosis, and most people monitor this by using a blood test or urine strips.

Many people just recommend the Keto diet for children who have epilepsy because getting rid of a complete food group will drastically change the way you eat, and this might pose some risks. Some evidence suggests that it might help adults who have epilepsy, too. Be careful as there needs to be more research done.

If this diet isn't followed properly and safely, the Keto diet could cause an increased risk of kidney stones and possible heart disease, as well as deficiencies in essential vitamins and minerals. Until your body gets adapted, the buildup of Ketones could cause mental fatigue, bad breath, nausea, and headaches.

You probably will lose some weight with both of these diets. At first, it will just be water weight. There is a chance that water weight might be regained when you begin eating normally again. Studies show that people who followed the Atkins diet lost 4.6 to 10.3 pounds, though they did regain some back by the end of their second year.

Neither the Atkins nor Keto diet makes you count calories. The main thing to make sure of is that you stay under the number of net carbs. Keto does recommend you to be sure you are hitting the right percentage of calories that come from fat and protein.

It all depends on the person as to which diet is the easiest for them to follow. It just depends on your habits before you start this diet. Neither one of them is easy.

The biggest difference between these two diets is the amount of protein you get to eat. Atkins doesn't put a cap on your protein consumption but Keto does. The other difference is having your body in Ketosis during the entire diet. The Keto diet is the only one that requires you to stay in Ketosis. The Atkins diet lets you slowly reintroduce carbs.

This means that the Atkins diet might be a bit more sustainable in the long run since it isn't as restrictive.

A Doctor's Point of View

According to leading cardiologist Dr. Ibal Sebag the Keto diet is a healthy way to lose weight. It is also an effective way to help with some diseases, if it is done the right way and with the help of a qualified health professional. This diet isn't for everybody—and this is why it is recommended to seek the advice of a dietitian or your doctor before beginning the Keto diet. If it was easy to eat nutritious foods and only the number of calories we need to keep us healthy, there wouldn't be diabetes or obesity epidemic. Many people have claimed they have tried every diet out there, and the Keto diet was the only one that worked for them because of the reduced cravings for high carb, processed, and sugary foods. Carry excess weight around the stomach area can increase a person's risk of developing health problems like depression, cancers, sleep apnea, osteoarthritis, stroke, heart disease, and diabetes. For people who have these risks, finding a diet that works is very important.

If you already follow the Keto diet here are some things that Dr. Sebag recommends you do:

1. Talk with a dietitian to make sure your micronutrient requirements are being met. Low carb and high-fat foods often have low water content, antioxidants, fiber, minerals, and vitamins. You have to be careful or you might risk dehydration, electrolyte imbalance, constipation, and vitamin deficiencies. A dietitian will be able to work with you to make sure you are eating the correct foods.

2. Before beginning the Keto diet, talk with your doctor. Get blood work done and know if you are at risk for cardiovascular disease. Your team of doctors can work together to help you achieve your diet and health care goals safely.

3. Try to eat mostly healthy fats such as olive oil, fatty fish, avocados, seeds, and nuts. You need to limit saturated fats.

4. Try to eat vegetables and fruits from every color group each day. Meaning you need to focus on more vegetables than fruits. Look for vegetables that are red, blue/purple, yellow/orange, white/brown, and green. Having a variety of colors will help guard against deficiencies in micronutrients. Make sure you include some foods that contain soluble fiber, legumes, raw nuts, and unsweetened cocoa powder.

5. Stay hydrated. Drink a lot of water. This is an absolute must.

Chapter 1: Ketogenic Lifestyle

Have your friends invited you to go out? Are you afraid to go with them due to food choices?

... Well, you don't have to be. You can eat delicious foods wherever you go.

- Add more good fats.

  Eating at restaurants can be difficult because their meals are usually low in fats. This makes it hard to feel full when you aren't eating carbs. You can handle this in a number of different ways. Ask for some extra butter, and melt it over your vegetables or meat. Ask for vinegar and olive oil-based dressing for salads. Many restaurants serve cheap vegetable oils that are high in omega 6 fatty acids instead of olive oil. People who have been doing the Keto diet will carry a small bottle of olive oil with them.

- Choose drinks wisely.

  The best drinks to choose are unsweetened tea, sparkling water, coffee, and water. If you want to drink alcoholic beverages, stick to dry wine, champagne, or spirits. Ask for them either with club soda (no sugar) or straight.

- Restaurants

  There are many restaurants along with fast food places that offer low-carb options. If you are craving a burger, ask for it to be wrapped in lettuce or leave the bun off. Choosing meats such as steak and fish will keep you in low-carb mode. Never choose any type of potato, rice or beans as a side. And instead, ask for salads, asparagus, and veggies. If you have a Chipotle near you, you can ask for a bowl without rice or beans and have it filled with cheese, meat, sour cream, and guacamole.

- Avoid starchy foods.

Say no to potatoes, pass the bread, bounce on the pasta, and flick the rice. Never allow temptations to get on your plate. Make sure you order your meal without any starchy sides.

When ordering an entrée, many places will let you substitute starchy sides for a salad or extra vegetables. When ordering a sandwich or burger, ask for it to be wrapped in lettuce instead of the bread. If the place won't make any substitutes, don't order the item at all.

If it does get on your plate, figure out your options. If you know you can leave it on your plate without eating it, go for it. If you can't handle the temptation, ask your waiter to replace it with a nonstarchy food. If the place is a casual restaurant, you can just throw it away.

- Be careful with sauces and condiments.

  Sauces contain mostly fats which is okay, however you need to be aware that gravies and ketchup contain mainly carbs. If you don't know what is in a sauce, ask your server what is in it and stay away from them if it has sugar or flour. You could ask them to put the sauce on the side so you can decide how much you want to add.

- Buffets

  This is when things can get tricky. Set some ground rules before you leave the table. Stay away from starches and grains. Go for fats, veggies, and protein.

- Dessert

  If you aren't hungry, ask for a cup of coffee or tea while waiting for your companions to finish. If you are still a bit hungry, see if they have some berries with whipped cream or a cheese plate.

Now that we've covered about what to do when you go out to eat, let's look at the top five restaurants that are Keto-friendly and what you can order.

1. Number Five – Chick-Fil-A

   Chick-fil-A has many low-carb options, especially breakfast. You can get a Keto sandwich and a coffee, and you will be energized until lunch. The grilled chicken nuggets are flavorful but they do have fillers and two carbs per eight nuggets.

   Their avocado lime ranch dressing has three grams of carbs and 32 grams of fat that comes from soybean oil. You might want to stay away from vegetable oil since they can increase inflammation and are full of trans fats.

   Here is a list of their Keto options:

   - Grilled chicken nuggets with a side salad
   - Grilled chicken club sandwich without the bun
   - Grilled chicken sandwich without the bun
   - Bacon, egg, and cheese muffin without the muffin
   - Sausage, egg, and cheese biscuit without the biscuit
   - Bacon, egg, and cheese biscuit without the biscuit

2. Number Four – Kentucky Fried Chicken

   Order your chicken grilled when visiting this restaurant. Their grilled chicken is delicious. You can choose a side with this meal, and their only Keto-friendly option is green beans. The grilled chicken is low in fat so add some fat like olive oil, butter, or avocado to make it filling. Watch out for the "butter" it is actually margarine.

   There are only two Keto options at this restaurant:

   - Green beans
   - Grilled chicken

3. Number Three – Jimmy John's Gourmet Sandwiches

Jimmy John's has a refreshing unwich. They offer a lettuce wrap instead of using bread, and it is really good. It isn't just a few lettuce leaves that are barely holding your fillings together. This is a favorite restaurant with the Keto crowd because their ingredients are fresh and simple.

Here is a list of their Keto-friendly Unwiches:

- Club tuna
- Beach club
- Country club
- Smoked Ham
- Ultimate porker
- Club Lulu
- Bootlegger club
- Hunters club
- Italian nightclub
- Billy club

Ask for a jumbo kosher dill pickle for your side.

4. Number Two – Chipotle

Chipotle is a great Keto restaurant. Their salad bowl comes with lettuce instead of beans and rice, and there is a multitude of options that can be put on top. Try to stay away from their vinaigrette as it is full of sugar. For a creamier kick, add sour cream or queso. If you don't have a Chipotle around and want Mexican, go to Taco Bell and order the Mini Skillet Bowl.

Here is a list of their Keto-friendly toppings:

- Guacamole
- Cheese
- Tomatillo-red chili salsa
- Tomatillo greed chili salsa

118

- Fresh tomato salsa
- Fajita vegetables
- Sofritas
- Chorizo
- Barbacoa
- Port carnitas
- Steak
- Chicken
- Romaine lettuce

5. Number One – Wendy's

You might not be a fan of fast food burgers, but Wendy's burgers are 100 percent all beef. They don't contain any fillers and are bigger than normal fast food burgers. The ingredients are as good as if you made everything at home.

Here are all the Keto options you can find here:

- Caesar side salad – without croutons
- Southwest avocado chicken salad
- Berry burst chicken salad – instead of ordering raspberry vinaigrette order Caesar or ranch dressing
- Grilled Asiago ranch chicken club sandwich – without the bun
- Grilled chicken sandwich – without honey mustard
- Cheesy cheddar burger – without the bun
- Jr. Bacon cheeseburger – without the bun
- Jr. Hamburger deluxe – without ketchup
- Cheeseburger deluxe – without bun or ketchup
- Bacon deluxe ¾ pound triple – without the bun
- Bacon deluxe ½ pound double – without the bun
- Bacon deluxe ¼ pound single – without the bun
- Son of baconator – without the bun
- Baconator – without the bun
- Dave's triple – without the bun
- Dave's double – without the bun
- Dave's single – without the bun

119

Five Common Mistakes On The Keto Diet

Looking at It as Just Another Fad Diet

After you have figured out why you want to do the Keto diet, you will need to seriously think about how realistic it will be for your lifestyle. You might need to manage an illness, lose some weight, or fuel for running.

Living the Keto Lifestyle has to be an all or nothing mindset. When you think about the entire system, it is a lot more than just cutting out sugar and bread for a week or so to get your body into Ketosis. It could take from a few weeks to a month for your body to begin using fat for fuel. Your body's natural instinct is to use sugar for its fuel. All your hard work and sacrifice can be undone with just one meal. Keto isn't a diet you can do just during the week and eat whatever you want on the weekends.

If you are using Keto to help you lose weight and restrict your calories, you might regain all of your lost weight if you go off Keto. This holds true if you use Keto to keep you from overeating foods such as cookies and pizza because you are going to overeat these when you decide to stop doing Keto.

If thinking about Keto as a new lifestyle doesn't seem like something you would enjoy, it isn't going to work for you.

Still Consuming Carbs

You may think you have been cutting out carbs, but the truth is they can creep into your diet and knock you out of Ketosis. This happens when you don't measure your portions, aren't keeping track of your carbs, or eat something without looking at the ingredients. Certain supplements and medicines could even up your intake of carbs.

When doing Keto right, it means your intake of carbs per day should be 20 grams or less. To keep you in this range, your carbs need to come from cauliflower, broccoli, and leafy greens. Even these veggies can add up if you aren't careful. One cup of kale has around five grams of net carbs. A kale salad, on the other hand, will weigh in at 20 grams because there are about three or four cups of kale in that salad.

One-fourth of a cup of sweet potatoes has 20 grams of carbs, and one medium apple has 23. Either one of these can max out your carbs for the day.

Incorrectly Managing Your Vegetables

When you think about the issue of carbs, keeping a balanced vegetable intake with this diet is very tricky. When you take the high carb foods such as quinoa, beans, lentils, and sweet potatoes off the table, you are going to have to be creative to build a diet that is balanced with foods that you can eat. If you get rid of all vegetables and concentrate on fat intake, you are leaving yourself open for deficiencies in minerals and vitamins.

To keep your diet nutritious, find your ten most favorite vegetables and look up their net carb content to see if you can put them into your new lifestyle. Try to add leafy greens that are full of nutrients such as spinach and kale into each meal. Always use a food tracker to keep track of your carb intake and watch out for portion sizes. To help with gaps in nutrients, you might want to think about taking a multivitamin.

In the first weeks of doing a Keto diet, and you begin losing weight from water, your electrolyte level might drop, and you may feel a bit crappy. If you experience any muscle problems or fatigue, try taking a supplement such as potassium and magnesium. Avocados, kale, and spinach give you potassium. And oysters, spinach, and hemp seeds will giveyou're your magnesium.

Consuming Large Amounts of Protein

Many fitness enthusiasts and healthy eaters talk about the benefits of a high protein diet, however too much protein is a big no-no with a Keto diet. When you eat too much protein, your body will turn it into glucose, and this can knock you out of Ketosis and back into burning sugar

Keto lets you eat a moderate intake of protein which is about 0.5 to .075 grams of protein for each pound of your body weight each day. If you weigh at 150 pounds this would equal to about 75 to 112 grams of protein every day. Three eggs or a small piece of chicken gives you 20 grams of protein.

Even though you are loading up on fats, you still need to take care of your heart. Protein needs to come from sources such as fish, turkey, and chicken instead of processed foods.

Consuming the Wrong Fats

When you need fat to take up around 80 percent of your total calorie intake, it is way too easy to add butter or coconut oil to everything you put in your mouth. Eating the correct types and maintaining a balance of fats is the key to a healthy Keto diet.

It is critical to get lots of unsaturated fats. Eating fatty foods such as sardines, trout, and salmon; avocados, seeds such as hemp, chia, and flax; and nuts such as pecans, walnuts, and peanuts are all good sources of unsaturated fats. Plant oil such as hemp oil, grapeseed, flax, and avocado are also good sources of unsaturated fats. Unsaturated fats can help reduce the risk of stroke and heart disease.

Self-Discipline and Willpower

There are millions of people out there who want to lose weight. Their biggest challenge is having a lack of self-discipline or willpower. Most people think they can't lose weight because they don't have any self-control. Whatever way you would like to define it, self-control, self-discipline, or willpower is a mysterious and elusive thing. Since the early 1960s, scientists have tried to figure out what self-discipline and willpower is and ways to improve it. People always complain that if they had more self-control they could avoid alcohol, drugs, eat better, exercise more, lose weight, eat more bacon, save for retirement, stop procrastinating, etc. One study showed that around 30 percent of the people they interviewed said their greatest barrier was their lack of willpower when making changes in their lives.

Excellence is a habit.

Excellence has never been an act. It has always been a habit of repetitive action. In order to understand self-discipline and willpower, you need to understand habit. Habits get created because our brains are always looking for ways to conserve energy. If left alone, our brains would take anything we do and make a habit out of it. It does this to conserve energy and effort. This lets us keep from thinking about normal everyday behaviors such as eating and walking so we can use our mental fuel for more important things such as designing video games, building airplanes, finding bacon, or making weapons.

Our brains will make time-saving patterns during its thought processes in the same way water reacts to dirt. When you drop water onto a mound of dirt, the water will run off to the side to find the path of least resistance. Every drop will erode a small channel down the side. The more water you drop, the deeper each channel will be carved on this hill. After some time, the water will run down that same channel over and over. In order for the water to go down this channel, the water has to be dropped on the top of the channel. This starting point is its trigger. When the water hits the trigger, it will always go along the same channel. Always.

Habits are our thought channels.

It takes a lot of effort to make water run out of that channel. This is just like our habits. Habits are impulse channels inside our brain that will follow a specific past that leads to the exact same outcome each time without any effort. All this is needed is a trigger. This impulse will follow the channel in our brain without creating a physical or mental routing to happen that will lead to a reward. This is called a habit loop. Basically, your brain has created a trigger that leads to a routine that leads to a reward.

Willpower—what is it?

What exactly is self-discipline and willpower? It's the ability to stay away from unproductive thought patterns. To redirect this habit will take a lot of mental energy. The first studies about willpower give the impression that willpower is a learned skill.

To quote Henry P. Liddon: "What we do upon some great occasion will probably depend on what we already are, and what we are will be the result of previous years of self-discipline." This basically meant that self-control can either be improved or learned. When you repeat a task over and over, it will get easier and take less effort. Therefore, excellence is not an act but a habit of repetition.

This in no way explains why we eat healthy one day and the next; we raid the refrigerator and eat everything in sight. You might be able to exercise on a day without any problems, but the next you can't get out of the bed. Exercising each day wouldn't be hard to do if it was a skill. The problem with the theory of self-discipline is you can't forget a skill.

Willpower is a muscle.

One researcher, Mark Muraven figured out that willpower is more similar to a muscle. He wanted to figure out if willpower were a skill, why can't it stay constant daily?

An experiment was conducted by putting a plate of fresh-baked cookies beside a bowl of radishes. They place the bowls on a table. This closet was set up with a two-way mirror, a toaster oven, a bell, and a chair. They asked for 67 student volunteers and instructed them to skip one meal. Each student filed into the room and sat down at the two bowls. A researcher instructed them that the experiment was about taste perception. This experiment was forcing the student to exert their self-discipline and willpower.

Researchers instructed half of the volunteers to ignore the radishes and eat the cookies. The other half were told to ignore the cookies and eat the radishes. The theory was that it was going to take willpower and mental energy to ignore cookies. It wasn't going to take any energy whatsoever to ignore the radishes when you are staring at a plate full of warm cookies.

The instructor reminded them they could only eat the food they were assigned and left them in the room.

After only five minutes, the volunteers who were allowed to eat cookies were in absolute heaven. The volunteers who were told to eat the radishes were experiencing mental agony.

One researcher reported that one radish eater grabbed a handful of cookies, ate them quickly, and licked any remaining chocolate off their fingers. Another picked up a cookie, smelled it, and placed it back onto the plate. After only five minutes, the radish eater's willpower has been completely exhausted by having to eat a bad tasting vegetable and ignoring a treat. Cookie eaters didn't use any self-discipline at all.

Researchers then went into the room and had the volunteers wait for 15 minutes to allow time for the sensory memory of the food they ate to diminish. In order to pass the time, they were asked to complete a simple puzzle. They were told to trace a shape without lifting their pencil or tracing over a line twice. If they wanted to quit, the researcher left a bell for them to ring. The researcher told them the puzzle shouldn't take them too long to complete. The truth was, the puzzle was impossible to do.

This was the most important part of the experiment. It took great amounts of willpower to continue working on the puzzle, especially after every attempt lead to failure.

What they realized behind their mirror was the cookies eaters had a large reserve of willpower and worked more than 30 minutes on the puzzle even after hitting all the roadblocks.

The radish-eaters with their depleted willpower grumbles showed frustration and complained. Some of them went so far as to shut their eyes and lay their heads down on the desk. One particular person snapped at the researcher when they came back into the room. The radish-eaters only averaged about eight minutes. When they were asked how they felt, one went so far as to say they were completely sick of this dumb experiment.

Cookie Fatigue

When they forced the volunteers to use their self-discipline and willpower to ignore the cookies, it put them in a state of wanting to quit a lot faster. Over 200 studies have been done since this one, and all of them found the same results — willpower is similar to a muscle. It isn't a skill. Willpower can fatigue a person.

This might be why people who choose to have an extramarital affair usually begin them at night after working all day. It is the reason behind why good doctors make stupid mistakes after a long complicated task has taken a lot of intense focus. It is also the reasons why most people will lose control when drinking or cheating on their diet.

Many people feel as if they have no willpower. Self-control and willpower are both learned behaviors that will happen with time. They are also very affected by fatigue. Anybody can have willpower. You have to know how it can be strengthened and weakened.

Intelligence isn't as important as willpower.

One study done in 2005 showed that when it comes to academic success, self-discipline and willpower were more important than how intelligent a person was. It also showed that having better self-discipline lead to less alcoholism, better relationships, higher grades, better self-esteem, and less binge eating. This is great.

Willpower does get stronger the more you use it but has no shelf life. It has to be used daily. It is always stronger during the beginning of the day. It will decline throughout the day as you get more tired.

Ways to Improve This Muscle

The first thing you have to do is write down the motivation or reasons why you want to change. This change must end at a goal. Wanting to lose weight isn't good enough. You need to be motivated due to the consequence of being overweight. Again losing weight isn't a clear goal. You need to set a certain weight you want to get to. You need to write it down legibly along with your reason. For example, "I will lose 50 pounds to help prevent me from getting diabetes." This is a great goal. Self-control and willpower can't happen until these other steps happen. Writing a goal along with two specifics and reading that goal every day will create a trigger by giving the goal specifics.

The next thing you need to do is monitor how you act toward the goal. When trying to lose weight, you need to keep a diet journal. You will need to write down every single thing you drink and eat. Each evening, write out your plan for the next day's meals. That evening, you will audit yourself for either your failures or successes by writing on the same page what you really did drink and eat. Keep doing the same routine every evening. You have to be honest with yourself about why you either failed or succeeded. This last part is what is very powerful. It is called self-introspection. This is the key that lets you see your habits. You will be able to make changes and get rid of any bad habits you see. This helps you strengthen your willpower and form good habits.

Willpower will get strengthened and developed with time. It gets developed by holding yourself accountable for every little thing every day. It has to be written down. If you plan on eating eggs and bacon for breakfast, and you chose something else—why? When you can look at your day, you might realize that you went to bed later than usual and that you didn't get up early enough to cook. So, you choose a yogurt that was readily available in the refrigerator. If you want to have eggs and bacon the next day you have to either fix them the night before, go to bed earlier, or get rid of the yogurt so it won't be a temptation. Planning will reinforce the trigger and gets rid of the mental energy that is needed to have willpower when you don't get enough sleep, feeling too stressed for getting up late, or not having any bacon. It can also give you more willpower to make better decisions during your day. Planning and writing down the next day's tasks gives you strength for willpower in the future and gets rid of fatigue that is needed to make changes the next day.

With time, self-introspection will get easier. It will get to a point that you will do it without even thinking about it. It is the subconscious self-introspection that gets seen by others as willpower and self-control. It is just like exercising to strengthen muscles, writing down small goals and making yourself accountable will make your self-discipline stronger. This self-discipline muscle will get very powerful. With time, you are going to be able to make decisions without really thinking about them. Your stronger willpower will be seen by people around you. You will see that you are just flexing a very well rested self-discipline muscle.

Now you need to attack the hardest decisions during your day in the mornings when you are more energized. These are the things that take the most energy. This gives you more strength to keep your willpower. During the evenings, when your willpower is weak, have some good snack available so you won't be tempted to cheat. Macadamia nuts, guacamole, pork rinds, some pre-cooked bacon, hard cheeses, or rolled meats are all good choices. Learn to make fat bombs and have them handy in the fridge will give you a boost of energy to make better choices when thinking about what you will fix for supper.

Chapter 2: Transitioning to a Keto Diet

You may have seen the word macros when researching the Keto diet but don't have any idea what they are. Well, "Macros" is just short for macronutrients when used in the context of the Keto diet.

Macros are the parts of food that give you fuel and energy. These are protein, carbohydrates, and fats. Your calories come from these. You need to grasp the concept of macros if you want to have a successful Keto diet. They have to be in balance to keep you in Ketosis.

Carbs are the only macro that you don't need to eat to keep you alive. There are essential fatty acids and amino acids. These are the building blocks of fats and proteins. There aren't any essential carbohydrates.

Carbs are made up of two things—sugars and starches. Fiber is looked at as a carb, but while doing a Keto diet, it isn't counted toward your total carb intake. The main reason fiber doesn't get counted is because our bodies don't digest fiber, so it doesn't have any effects on our blood sugar.

This means when you look at a nutrition label, you need to first look for the total carbs and then look for fiber. You need to subtract the amount of fiber from the total number of carbs, and this gives you your net carb count.

Total carbs – fiber = net carbs

This basically means that net carbs only count the sugars and starches in the carbohydrates. When you figure up your macros for a meal, you only use net carbs. You don't use total carbs.

In order for you to succeed, you need to find foods that are naturally low in carbs and the ones that aren't. They aren't going to be obvious. It is obvious that potatoes are high in carbs but did you know that bananas are also high in carbs?

For anyone starting a Keto diet, you need to try and consume about 20 grams of net carbs daily.

Protein is important to our bodies because it will help preserve lean muscle mass, makes hormones and enzymes, the energy source in the absence of carbs, growth, tissue repair, and immune function. Protein plays an important role in our biological processes. Proteins are called the building blocks in a healthy body.

When we eat these, they get broken down into amino acids. Nine of these can't be produced by our bodies. This is why these essential amino acids need to come from our food. These nine includes tryptophan, valine, phenylalanine, threonine, lysine, leucine, histidine, methionine, isoleucine. If there is a deficiency in protein or any of these amino acids, it could cause kwashiorkor, malnutrition, or any other health problems.

When you follow a Keto diet, you need to be sure you eat enough protein to help preserve your lean body mass. The amount you need to eat all depends on your current amount of lean body mass. Here is a guideline:

- 0.7 to 0.8 grams of protein per pound of muscle to help preserve your muscle mass.
- 0.8 to 1.2 grams of protein per pound of muscle to help you increase your muscle mass.

You don't ever want to lose a body mass. You should only gain or preserve. Many people only focus only on losing weight. Many times losing weight mean losing muscle along with fat. Your goal needs to be losing fat and saving your muscles. This is important for people to keep good metabolism.

The main thing is making sure you don't get crazy when you eat protein while following a Keto diet. Too much might put too much stress on your kidneys and could affect Ketosis. Try keeping your macros in the ranges above.

Here is an example:

Let's say you weigh 160 pounds and you have 30 percent body fat. This means you have about 48 pounds of body fat. Then you subtract your body fat from your total weight and this gives you your lean body mass. For this example, it would be 112 pounds.

To figure out how much protein you need to eat, you have to take the lean body mass number and multiply it by the ration from earlier. For this example, you need to eat 89.6 grams of protein every day to preserve your muscle mass. Here is how it looks when written down:

112 pounds of muscle x 0.8 grams of protein = 89.6 grams

The last macro is fat. We need to eat a good amount of fat to help maintain cell membranes, provide protection for organs, absorb specific vitamins, development, energy, and growth. These fats will also help you feel fuller longer.

Dietary fats will get broken down into fatty acids and glycerol. This body can't synthesize two types of fatty acids, so it is very important that you eat them. These fatty acids are linoleic acid and linoleic acid.

These fats are satiating, so it's great for people who want to fight off hunger pangs. Now you need to figure how much fat you need to consume. If your carbs at a minimum, you've already figured out how much protein you should eat, and then the rest of your dietary needs are met with fat.

To maintain your weight, you will eat enough calories from fat to support your regular expenditure. If you want to burn fat, then you will need to eat in a deficit.

You have been given a lot of information to help you figure out your macros, but there is an easier way to figure this out. You can find many different online calculators to help you figure out these numbers without getting a headache. If you would like to use an online calculator, check out the website *Ketogains*. Theirs works great.

Now, if you would like to figure this out on your own, let's continue with the 160 pounds from earlier. Let's say this person is a female, stands 5'4", in her late 20s, and has a desk job. She is mainly sedentary.

Let's plug her into the calculator:

The base metabolic rate would be 1467 kcal.

Daily energy expenditure would be 1614 kcal.

She needs to eat about 90 grams of protein, 20 grams of net carbs, and 86 grams of fat. Her intake is made up of 72 percent fat, 23 percent protein, and 5 percent carbs.

Now you know what macros are and how to figure out your numbers. You are on your way to getting started with a Keto diet.

Foods You Need to Stay Away From

- Sugar – this is the big no-no. You need to stop drinking soft drinks, sports drinks, fruit juices, and vitamin water. Also:

    - Frozen treats
    - Candy
    - Breakfast cereals
    - Sweets
    - Donuts
    - Cakes
    - Chocolate bars
    - Cookies

- Starches:

    - Lentils

- Porridge
- Bread
- Muesli
- Pasta
- Potato chips
- Rice
- French fries
- Potatoes
- Sweet potatoes
- Beans

- Fruit

- Margarine – you need to use real butter and none of the fake kind.

- Beer – this is nothing but liquid bread.

- Pre-packaged low-carb foods – be sure you read the label before you purchase any of these. Atkins products are not all low-carb.

Trickiest Hidden Carbs

Carbs can be hidden anywhere. Many people think that if you cook your meals and stay away from processed foods, you can say away from all hidden carbs. This isn't true. You might be making tacos at home, including chips and salsa, you are still racking up the exact same carbs as if they were bought from a fast food restaurant.

Hidden carbs like to hide in healthy options such as sugar-free foods.

- Sugar alternatives/alcohols

Sugar alcohols or "the polyols," are in anything that is labeled sugar free or carb free. They aren't zero-carb and some can cause insulin spikes or increased blood sugar levels.

- Molasses

- Yacon syrup
- Agave
- Honey
- Vegetable glycerin
- Spenda
- Maltitol
- Sorbitol
- Xylitol

You can use Erythritol, pure liquid sucralose, or stevia.

- Sauces and Seasonings

You know how to stay away from sweet sauces, but there are other flavorings that can quickly add up to your daily carb count and might be the source of uncalculated carbs. It doesn't matter how delicious and "healthy" these are.

Here is a list of carbs that are in spices, herbs, sauces, and seasonings:

In one tablespoon:

- Paprika – 3.3 grams
- Cayenne – 3 grams
- Oregano – 3.3 grams
- Chili powder – 4.1 grams
- Onion powder – 5.4 grams
- Garlic powder – 6 grams
- Ground cumin – 2.75 grams

Ground/dried less than one grams per teaspoon:

- Coriander
- Black pepper
- Cloves
- Ginger
- Cinnamon
- Basil

- Mint
- Tarragon

Blended spices about one gram per teaspoon:

- Bouillon powders or cubes: one gram per ½ cube
- Pie Spice
- Garam masala
- Chinese 5-spice
- Curry powder
- Any other blended spices just read the label carefully. Look at larger containers if they small ones don't have the information

Fresh

- Lime/lemon juice: 1 gram per tablespoon
- Lime/lemon rind: 1 gram per teaspoon
- Garlic: 1 large clove or 1 teaspoon minced: 1 gram
- Ginger root: 1 gram per tablespoon

Hot sauces, soy sauce, vinegar

- Wine vinegar, cider, and white are all zero-carb.
- Balsamic vinegar: 2 grams per tablespoon
- Balsamic oil, plain: 3 grams per two tablespoons
- Balsamic oil, processed: 9 to 12 grams per two tablespoons
- Red hot or Tabasco sauce has zero carbs
- Soy sauce: .5 grams per teaspoon
- Jamaican, Trinidad, and Cajun read the label carefully.

Extracts or flavor concentrates:

- Orange

- Vanilla
- Almond
- All have .5 grams per teaspoon

Mayonnaise and mustard:

- Dijon or plain: less than .5 grams per teaspoon
- Real mayonnaise: .5 grams per tablespoon

- Protein Bars and Supplements

Anything that is flavored, chewable, or coated are going to be loaded with carbs. If you take two, you have already eaten seven grams of carbs before you ate breakfast. Protein bars are loaded with carbs.

Staying Hydrated

When you are doing a Ketogenic diet, your body will switch its fuel supply from glucose to fat. Insulin levels might become low and fat burning will increase drastically. It will become easy for your body to access your stored fat and then burn it. This is great when trying to lose weight, but there are other benefits, too.

You have to drink a lot of water to make sure you stay hydrated.

Dehydration could cause many problems such as fatigue, cramps, and headaches. Water is extremely important in allowing good health and sustaining life.

Did you realize that it is recommended that you drink in ounces half of your body weight in pounds? Let's say you weigh 160 pounds. This means you need to drink 80 ounces of water each day.

When following a Keto diet, your body will retain less water, gets rid of large amounts of sodium, and your insulin sensitivity will increase. This could cause dehydration.

When your body is getting rid of all the stored glucose it is also losing water. This is why you need to replenish all the water you lose.

- Side Effects of Dehydration

  When you are hydrated, it allows your body to get rid of all toxins that enter your body. Dehydration can build up toxins and this can cause many health problems.

  Mild dehydration could cause dry skin, dizziness, fatigue, and headaches. When you are taking a long car trip, children don't seem to drink the right amount of water. Yes, this might mean you have to stop more frequently for potty breaks but it is better than your children feeling dizzy and possible fainting.

  Severe dehydration could cause major problems such as rapid heartbeat, fever, low blood pressure, and confusion.

- Symptoms of Dehydration

  It isn't always easy to know when you are dehydrated. You need to listen to your body so you can avoid dehydration. Here are some ways you might notice it:

1. The color of your urine: When you look at the color of your urine, you will be able to see if your body needs water. If your urine is darker than the color of a dandelion, it might mean you need to drink more water. Ideally you want your urine to be clear of light, light yellow.

2. Dry mouth or lips: If you notice your mouth is drier than normal, this is telling you your body needs more water.

- How to Prevent Dehydration

  There are several ways you can prevent dehydration:

1. Eat vegetables that are high in water like lettuce, greens, and celery. These could help you become more hydrated. Try to include these in your daily vegetables.

2. Stay away from drinks and foods that promote dehydration: Foods that are high in sodium will cause you to feel dehydrated. Because you are going to be eating more foods with higher sodium content during the Keto diet, it is extremely important to drink lots of water.

3. Coffee: This is a diuretic and could cause dehydration if you drink too much. Adding cream and butter will help increase your fat consumption.

4. Watch out for activities that might cause dehydration: exercising, hiking, walking, running, and other activities that will make you sweat. This removes water from your body and makes hydrating yourself very important.

5. Remain hydrated through the day: You need to create a habit of drinking water more often. It is about you taking care of your health and body. If you have to make a chart that shows eight cups of water and check them off as you drink them. Drink water even if you don't feel thirsty.

Here are some tips to increase hydration through drinking water:

- At home:
    - When you get up every day
    - Before a meal
    - After meals
    - After finishing a chore

- On the go:
    - Each hour when on a long trip
    - Driving home from work or after taking children to school
    - Driving to work or running errands

- At work:
  - Before and after meetings
  - During break times

- When flying:
  - Before meals
  - After meals
  - Every hour or so

Here are some ways you can motivate yourself to stay hydrated:

- Add lemon juice to water
- Drink green tea
- Keep water with you at all times
- Drink your water warm if you don't like cold water

When you drink enough water you are going to:

- Help manage your weight
- Keeps your body from getting overheated
- Aids in digestion
- Prevents constipation
- Gets rid of waste through urination and sweat
- Lubricated joints
- Keeps you alert
- Improves concentration
- Keeps your mind sharp
- Reduces headaches

Chapter 3: Apps To Count Your Intake

If you were to ask a group of people who have been following the Keto diet how they keep track of their macros, you are probably going to get different answers. We are going to be looking at two of the most popular apps that are out there. We will talk about how to use each one to track your macros as well as the pros and cons of each. It's important to realize you do not need an app to live Keto, its just helps and makes your life a lot easier.

MyFitnessPal

This is the most popular app out there. It is free if you don't want any of the extra features. This app put an emphasis on social networking and sharing your progress with friends. It also has a huge food database. Basically, any food you eat can be found on this app. Anybody who uses this app can add foods, and this makes it hard to know what food you should choose in their database.

This app doesn't track net carbs. This makes it harder for Keto dieters to use since you have to figure out your own net carbs.

Here are some pros and cons:

Pros:

- Tracking packaged foods that have barcodes
- Large food database
- Social sharing
- Option to add recipes from websites
- Weight gain/loss chart

Cons:

- Doesn't track net carbs
- Inaccurate food database
- Pop up advertisements in the app

- Only uses percentages and not grams

Cronometer

This app costs $2.99. The main differences between the two are the social media and the food database. Its food database is more accurate as it only lists validated entries with details such as amino acids and micronutrients. It app doesn't have to social sharing unless you buy the gold subscription. It does track net carbs where MyFitnessPal doesn't.

Here is a list of pros and cons:

Pros:

- Can interchange micronutrient and macronutrient goals by percentages and grams
- No ads
- Ketogenic diet mod with a net carb tracker
- Better precise food database

Cons:

- Costs $2.99
- No weight gain/loss chart
- Limited food database

Exercising When Doing a Keto Diet

We all know that we have better health when we exercise. If you follow a Keto diet, we know that you will lose some weight. What will happen if you mix the two?

It would be reasonable to assume that when you combine the two it would take your health and weight loss to another level. The truth is a bit more complicated. Since you are already restricting your carbs, there are many changes that might happen and some could even affect your exercise performance.

When you restrict intake of carbs, you are limiting your muscle cells from getting any sugar. This is the fastest fuel source. When your muscles can't access sugar, this impairs their function. High intensity is any activity that lasts longer than ten seconds. The reason for this is that after ten seconds of max effort, the muscles begin to burn glucose for energy through a metabolic pathway known as glycolysis.

Fat and Ketones are not a good substitute for glucose when working out. It is only after you have been working out for two minutes that your body will shift into a metabolic pathway that will use your Ketones and fat.

When you restrict your intake of carbs, you are basically depriving your muscles' cells of sugar that they need to fuel the activities for high-intensity effort for ten seconds to two minutes. This means if you are following a Keto diet, it is going to limit your performance during certain exercises such as:

- Swimming or sprinting for more than ten seconds.
- Weight lifting for more than five reps each set using a weight that is heavy enough to bring you close to failure.
- High-intensity circuit training or interval training.
- Playing a sport that gives you minimal breaks like rugby, lacrosse, and soccer.

This isn't a comprehensive list but it gives you an idea of the kinds of exercises that your body has to use glycolysis for. Remember that the metabolic pathway timing all depends on each individual. There are some people that might maintain performance for 30 seconds without needing carbs.

It is also important that you eat the correct amount of fats and protein when you exercise while following a Keto diet.

Many health professionals, when designing a diet plan, will set the protein intake first Protein always gets top priority because it performs actions that carbs and fats can't. Protein also helps improve satiation, has a better thermic effect, and stimulates muscle synthesis better than other macronutrients. If you don't

143

eat enough protein, you will lose muscle mass and might eat more calories than you should.

If you want to keep your exercise routine or implement one, you need to make sure you eat the correct amounts of macros. Here are a few guidelines:

- Excess calories should come from fats and not protein or carbs.
- Be sure your calorie intake stays in a deficit of about 250 to 500 calories. This is not a priority. Many people don't worry about calories while following a Keto diet.
- Keep your protein intake to around one gram per pound of body weight.

The majority of us aren't athletes and adding in an exercise routine isn't going to be hard. Cardio doesn't require you to exercise at high intensities that require your body to burn sugar and glycogen to get results. You just need to bring up your heart rate and keep it there.

Cardio is a low to moderate intensity and a Keto diet won't impair your performance. You might realize you can work out longer without getting tired when you are in Ketosis.

Here are some examples of good cardio workouts:

- Running
- Aerobic training classes
- Recreational sports
- Swimming
- Circuit training
- Cycling
- Interval training classes

You need to remember that your strength and power might be decreased during these workouts due to carb restriction. If you just want a good cardiovascular workout, it is important that you push yourself to your max strength and power.

Chapter 4: Getting Started

It's important that you understand what foods you can and cannot eat on a Keto diet. Let's go over all of the food that you can eat.

- Meats – You can enjoy all unprocessed meats because they are all low in carbs. If you can afford it, try to buy grass-fed organic meats. Make sure you don't go crazy with meats, though. You are supposed to eat more fats.

- Fish and seafood – All fish, like meats, are a great option. Salmon is the best of both worlds because it's the perfect source of omega 3s.

- Eggs – These are the most versatile foods that you can eat on Keto because you can fix them in many different ways.

- High-fat sauces – These are great ways to get your fat intake, especially if you use coconut oil and butter.

- Above-ground vegetables – You have to make sure that you pick veggies that grow above the ground. The best ones to pick from are:

  - Spinach
  - Zucchini
  - Asparagus
  - Avocado
  - Broccoli
  - Kale
  - Green beans
  - Cauliflower
  - Brussels sprouts

- High-fat dairy – Butter is the best choice here. You should go with real butter and not a tub of margarine. Cheese is another good option. You can eat high-fat yogurts in moderation, however normal milk comes with too much sugar.

- Nuts – These are best eaten in moderation. Carbs can sneak up quickly.

- Berries – These should also be eaten in moderation.

- Water – This is one of the most important things you need to consume.

- Coffee – You either have to consume it black or add some coconut oil and butter.

- Tea – Make sure you don't add sugar.

- Bone broth – This will add electrolytes and nutrients.

Let's Go Shopping

Now that you know what you can eat, you're going to want to shop. Here is a shopping list to help you out, and it's even organized by section.

- Miscellaneous

  - Pork rinds
  - Olives
  - Beef jerky
  - Sugar-free and full-fat dressings
  - Salsa
  - Hot sauce
  - Apple cider vinegar
  - Mustard
  - Pickles – sugar-free
  - Nut Flours
  - Nut butter
  - Nuts
  - Seeds
  - Oils

- Dairy

  - Heavy cream
  - Cheeses
  - Cream cheese
  - Eggs
  - Butter
  - High fat yoghurt

- Fruits

  - Avocados
  - Strawberries
  - Raspberries
  - Blackberries

- Vegetables

  - Zucchini
  - Squashes
  - Garlic
  - Onions
  - Lettuce
  - Broccoli
  - Cauliflower
  - Cabbage
  - Peppers
  - Cucumbers

- Fish

  - Salmon
  - Tuna
  - Shrimp

- Meats

- Ground beef
- Steaks
- Chicken
- Breakfast sausage
- Bacon
- Ground Pork
- Pork Chops
- Ham
- Hot dogs
- Deli Meats
- Pepperoni

Reading Food Labels

You will be finding yourself asking yourself, "Is this Keto?" a lot. We're going to quickly go over how to correctly read a food label so you don't get suckered in by hidden sugars.

First off, let me reiterate that you count net carbs: total carbs-dietary fiber. Alright, let's get started:

1. Read the ingredient list.

   Food manufacturers have to list their ingredients in order of weight. The heaviest is first and lightest is last. If starch or sugar is listed in the first five ingredients, stay away from it. The bad thing is that sugars come in many different names. Make sure you become familiar with sugars aliases.

   Bacon is a tricky one because it's hard to find one with sugar in the first five. There are three no-sugar options. Find brands that write "No Sugar Added" on the pack. Still read the ingredient to make sure they aren't lying. Head to the butcher and ask him to cut pork belly into bacon strips. If you have to pick one with added sugar, make sure the total carbs are zero.

2. What is the serving size?

Serving size is important so that you keep your net carb intake at the right level. Let's take cashews as an example. A serving size of cashews is supposed to be one ounce, which is around 18 pieces according to Google. If you ate those 18 pieces, you would be eating eight grams of carbs.

If you ate the whole bag of cashews, you would be eating 256 grams of carbs. That's way over 20 grams.

Total and net don't quite paint the entire picture because they don't really let you know how many carbs is actually in that container. That's why you have to look at the serving size and how many servings are in the container. This lets you know how much you can eat without going overboard.

Chapter 5: Benefits of the Keto Lifestyle

Anybody getting ready to start a new diet or lifestyle change is going to want to know all of the benefits that come along with it. Throughout this, you will learn about many different positive things that a Keto diet can bring. We are going to look, right now, at what all the hype is around the Ketogenic diet.

- Improves diabetes, obesity, and metabolic syndrome.

  This is the main reason why a lot of people will follow a Ketogenic diet. In all of the reasons we will look at, plus this reason, a Ketogenic diet is perfect for people who suffer from type 1 or type 2 diabetes. It is also perfect for people who are obese because it is able to help them burn off fat, and it spares muscle loss. The Keto diet is able to curb a lot of disorders that tend to happen because of obesity. This includes the symptoms and risk factors known as metabolic syndrome.

- It improves muscle endurance and muscle gain.

  It has been discovered that BHB helps promote muscle gain. When you combine this with a lot of anecdotal evidence through the years, a bodybuilder movement has happened with the Keto diet and how it can help them gain muscle. Ultra-endurance athletes started to use a Keto diet. After an athlete has become fat-adapted, evidence has suggested that their mental and physical performance has improved.

- It can improve eye health.

  The biggest problem that diabetics could end up facing is macular degeneration. It's common knowledge that high blood sugar can end up hurting a person's eyesight and can lead to a higher risk of cataracts. It shouldn't come as a surprise that when you lower your blood sugar levels, you will also improve your vision health and eyes.

- Can stabilize uric acid levels.

  The biggest culprit of gout and kidney stones are high levels of uric acid, calcium, oxalate, and phosphorus. The main cause of this is typically a combination of consuming things that have a lot of alcohol and purines, unlucky genetics, dehydration, obesity, and sugar consumption. The main caveat is that a Ketogenic diet can temporarily raise your uric acid levels, especially if you end up letting yourself become dehydrated. Over time, once you become adapted to the diet, and you make sure you consume enough water, your levels will lower.

- It helps fight against heart disease.

  A Ketogenic diet is able to lower blood pressure and triglyceride level and improve your cholesterol profiles. The reason for this is because of the effects of keeping blood glucose at a low and stable level. While it will likely sound counterintuitive that consuming more fat is going to lower your triglycerides, it has been discovered that too many carbs are the main reason for high triglyceride levels. When you look at HDL and LDL levels, a Keto diet can help raise your good cholesterol and to lower your bad cholesterol.

- Improve your sleep and energy.

  Once people reach day four or five of the diet, many of them report an increase in energy levels and fewer cravings for carbs. The main reason for this is, again, stable insulin levels and an energy source that is readily available for the brain and body tissues. It's still a mystery as to why it helps improve sleep. Studies have found that a

Keto diet helps sleep, as it decreases REM and increases slow-wave sleep patterns. The exact reason behind this is unclear; it probably has to do with the complex biochemical shifts involved in the brain using Ketones for energy combined with body burning fat.

Five Tips for Women

While the Keto diet stays the same for the most part no matter if you're a man or a woman, there are some gender-specific tips that can help you out. That's what the rest of the chapter is going to provide you with.

1. For the first week or so, eat extra fat

    This will do three things. First, it will upregulate your fat burning machinery. It helps your mitochondria to get used to a new fuel source.

    Second, it will make sure that you aren't working from a caloric deficit. It will let your body know you have plenty of food so that you won't go into a starvation mode.

    Third, it gives you a boost, psychologically. It helps you realize that you are able to eat more fat than you thought you could while still losing weight.

    You shouldn't keep eating all of the extra fat until you are trying to put on some weight. As your body gets used to burning Ketones, you can lower your fat intake.

2. Don't work to restrict your calorie intake.

    You know how a benefit of Keto is inadvertently restricting your calories? You shouldn't try to double down on the calorie restriction. Don't believe me. Allow yourself the first three weeks of Keto where you only track your macros. Make sure you are restricting your carbs, but don't keep track of anything else. Don't gorge yourself and don't melt a stick of butter into your coffee. Allow yourself to eat until you are full and then stop. You'll be surprised that you can still lose weight even if you don't track every little thing.

3. Keto and fasting, Remember that you can eat more Carbs.

   Even some men will suffer metabolically when they combine extreme low-carbs with intense fasting. Your calories can get too low for too long. You want to burn fat, but if your body gets too scared that you're not going to get any more food, it might hold onto your fat. By avoiding this , you can up your carbs 5-10%

4. Stay away from nutrient-poor fat bombs.

   Fat bombs are supposed to be your allies to help you through a tough time. Make sure that when you make fat bombs, you do so with the use of nutrient-dense foods. Better yet, grab a salad, olives, nut butter, an egg, and so on.

5. Don't be super strict.

   Making sure you strictly stick to the Keto diet for the first month is great to get you fat-adapted, but after that, you don't have to be so strict. You have created your fat-burning machinery. It's not going to kill you to enjoy a gluten-free cookie your kid surprises you with. Your body is going to bounce back at this point.

Five Tips for Men

1. Try intermittent fasting.

   This is a great way to keep yourself in Ketosis. It would be best to go low-carb and eat at regular times for a couple of days before you start fasting. This will prevent a hypoglycemic episode. This easiest way to fast is to skip breakfast.

2. Eat enough good salts.

For so long we have been told to reduce our sodium intake. But with a Keto diet, your kidneys will release more sodium which can cause a low sodium/potassium ratio. When you are on a Keto diet, you need to make sure that you get an additional three to five grams of sodium. A teaspoon of sea salt will give you around two grams of sodium.

Drinking broth during the day can help you out. Add extra sea salt to your meals is also a good idea. Sea veggies like nori and kelp have high salt content as well.

3. Make sure you exercise regularly.

   Regular exercising will help you activate the glucose transport molecule. This will help you adapt and maintain Ketosis because it will let you handle just a bit more carbs in the diet. Strength training exercises are a good idea and will improve receptor activity. Also, the greater amount of lean muscle you have, the more amount of fat you will burn.

4. Improve the motility of your bowels.

   Constipation is something that most people will face on Keto. Being constipated will knock you out of Ketosis. Eating more fermented foods, drinking a lot of water, adding more sea salt to your diet, and consuming more greens will help.

5. Don't consume too much protein.

   If you eat too much protein, and it would have to be a significant amount, your body can change it into glucose. This will knock you out of Ketosis. Make sure that your fat intake is higher than your protein intake, and everything should be okay.

Meal Plan and Keto on a Budget

A lot of people have the belief that Keto has to be expensive, but that's not true. Since you will be eating more fats, you will feel fuller for longer than you did on carbs, which means you won't eat as many meals. And not eating a bunch of snacks during the day will be its own money-saving tip.

Since you don't have to change your protein intake too much, you shouldn't have to buy a bunch of expensive meats. The following are some good money-saving tips for a Keto diet on a budget:

- Keep everything simple. You don't have to create meals with a bunch of working parts. The fewer ingredients that you cook with, the less money you are going to spend. A simple omelet with a side of water will probably cost you $3.50. A Big Mac would cost $5.

- Use the veggies and fruits that are in season. The rest of the year you can purchase frozen.

- Buying a whole chicken and cutting it apart on your own is usually cheaper. You can also keep the bones to make your own broth.

- Pay close attention to the deals that your supermarket is having and stock up on Keto-friendly items that are on sale, especially if it's something you use a lot of.

It's also a great idea to plan out your meals before you come up with your shopping list. This will keep you organized. Planning out your shopping trips is the best way to make sure you don't spend too much. When shopping, the following things can help you save money:

- Buy regular cheese. You don't need specialty cheeses. Buy in bulk and shred your own cheese at home.

- Skip packaged coleslaw. You can make your own for less.

- Go with simple meats and skip special ones.

- You don't have to get expensive kale. Choose the cheaper greens. They are just as nutritious.

- Cut out excessive nuts because they do add up.

- Pick almond meal instead of almond flour. You can also grind up your own almonds.

- Keep avocados to a minimum when they are out of season.

- Get frozen or canned fish, especially if you like salmon and tuna.

Get the best quality of foods that you are able to afford. Just because everybody believes you have to eat organic doesn't mean you have to. If you're not able to afford it, then do buy it. The main thing to remember is to cook your meals at home and they are going to be healthier, whether they're organic or not.

Also, pick the cheaper cuts of meats, and make sure you check on meats that have been marked down. Cooking all of your meals at home will also be cheaper than purchasing Keto-friendly meals at restaurants. Overall, it's not a big difference picking simple Keto recipes and not the fancy ones that require specialty ingredients.

Quick Meal Plan

Having a good idea of the meals you can eat can help you perform better on a Keto diet. Having options that are budget friendly are even better. Here, you will find nine different meal options separated between morning, lunch, and dinner. Three of these will be really easy on the budget.

Morning:

Bacon and Eggs (Budget Keto):
- 2 eggs

- 2 slices bacon
- Cherry tomatoes

Fry up the bacon and scramble the eggs and serve alongside a few cherry tomatoes.

Pizza Omelet:

- 2 slices bacon
- Basil, salt, pepper
- ½ oz. pepperoni slices
- .5 c shredded mozzarella
- 1 tbsp. heavy cream
- 3 eggs

Fry up the bacon. Beat the eggs, cream, pepper, basil, and salt together and pour into a preheated pan. Allow it to cook until almost done and then lay the pepperoni slices on top. Sprinkle with the cheese and fold the omelet in half. Allow it to cook for a moment and more and serve with the bacon.

Sausage, Egg, and Cheese with Coffee

- 2 oz. breakfast sausage
- 1 tbsp. olive oil
- Slice cheese
- Egg
- Bulletproof coffee

  - 1 tbsp. butter
  - 1 tbsp. coconut oil
  - 1 c hot coffee

Cook the egg sunny side up and cook the sausage in an oiled pan. Lay the sausage on a plate and top with the egg and cheese slice. Add the ingredients for the coffee to a blender and mix until frothy.

Lunch:

Keto Tuna Plate (Budget Keto):

- Pepper and salt
- Lemon
- .25 c mayonnaise
- .5 avocado
- 5 oz. tuna in oil
- 1 oz. baby spinach
- 2 eggs

Hard boil the eggs and let them cool in some ice water and then peel the eggs. Place the avocado, tuna, spinach, and eggs on a plate. Top with a dollop of mayo and a wedge of lemon.

Cobb Salad:

- 1 tbsp. olive oil
- .5 tsp white vinegar
- .25 avocado
- 2 slices bacon
- 4 oz. chicken
- Hard boil egg
- 1 c spinach

Cook the bacon and then chop up the cooked egg and bacon. Rip up the spinach leaves and top with the other ingredients. Dress with some low-carb bleu cheese or vinaigrette.

Bun-less Butter Burger:

- 1 tsp mayo
- 1 large lettuce leaf
- 1 tbsp. olive oil
- Slice cheese
- 1 tbsp. butter

- Paprika, salt, pepper
- 4 oz. ground beef

Add the seasoning to the ground beef and mix well. Form into two patties. Put the butter in the center of one patty and top with the other. Press together to seal the butter in. Cook until done. Place on a lettuce leaf, do top it with cheese, and do spread on some mayo.

Dinner:

Fried Cabbage with Crispy Bacon (Budget Keto):

- Pepper and salt
- 2 oz. butter
- 1 lb. green cabbage
- 10 oz. bacon

Chop up the bacon and cabbage. Fry the bacon until crispy. Add the butter and cabbage to the pan and cook until golden and soft. Season with some pepper and salt.

Chicken and Mushrooms:

- Handful of spinach
- Pepper, salt
- 1 tsp lemon juice
- .25 c heavy cream
- .25 c water
- 2 tbsp. butter
- 8 oz. mushrooms
- 6 oz. chicken

Add the chicken to a pan and cook until almost done. Allow it to rest as you cook the sauce. Add the butter and mushrooms to the pan, cooking until crisped up. Add in the cream, lemon juice, and water, cooking until thickened. Season with some pepper and salt. Nestle in the chicken and cook until done. Serve with the spinach.

10-Minute Pizza:

- Basil
- 2 tbsp. parmesan
- 1 oz. sliced pepperoni
- .5 c marinara sauce
- 1 c shredded mozzarella

Place half of the mozzarella in a pan. Allow it to cook and melt until browned. Pour in the sauce and spread around. Add on the pepperoni and the remaining cheese. Sprinkle with parmesan and enjoy.

Alcohol on Keto

Alcohol tends to come with a bad rap, and it is one of the most abused substances. It can also cause a big problem for people when dieting, but with self-control and moderation, it can be enjoyed.

If you like to enjoy a few beers, a few glasses of wine, or some shots on the weekends to relax or have a good time, then all is great. But toss in a low-carb diet, and you may find it hard. Most Keto followers will notice that their tolerance drops significantly after they start the diet. And once you find out your favorite drink has 30 grams of carbs, you may think about giving up alcohol altogether. You don't have to throw in the towel right away.

Alcohol can affect a diet in many ways. The first is the way it is metabolized. With a carb-rich diet, your body is busy breaking down sugars, so the alcohol is metabolized slower. On a low-carb diet, your glycogen stores are low and alcohol is metabolized right away. This is what makes you feel drunk.

Another problem with alcohol is that it lowers our inhibitions, which could cause mindless snacking and cheating. You might not realize what you've done until you wake up the next morning with a half of a pizza on your side.

There is also a problem with the fact that you may end up consuming alcohol on an empty stomach, which causes things to happen a lot faster. It's important that you reduce your alcohol consumption because it is just empty calories.

That all being said you are still able to enjoy alcohol in moderation on a Keto diet. Clear liquors at 40% alcohol are safe, and anything that tastes the least bit sweet isn't. Acceptable alcohols are:

- Cognac
- Brandy
- Scotch
- Rum
- Whiskey
- Gin
- Tequila
- Vodka

Wine and beer can still be enjoyed as well. However, you have to know which ones are lower in carbs. Try sticking to dry or semi-dry wines because they have the least amount of sugar. Carb and calorie content also differ based on the brand.

- Red wines:

  - Merlot – 3.7 carbs, 120 calories
  - Pinot noir – 3.4 carbs, 121 calories
  - Cabernet Sauvignon – 3.8 carbs, 120 calories

- White wines:

  - Champagne – 1.5 carbs, 96 calories
  - Riesling – 5.5 carbs, 118 calories
  - Chardonnay – 3.7 carbs, 118 calories
  - Sauvignon blanc – 2.7 carbs, 122 calories
  - Pinot Grigio – 3.2 carbs, 122 calories

There are plenty of low-carb beer options out there, too, if you look for them. Some good examples are:

- Bud light – 6.6 carbs, 110 calories

- Amstel light – 5 carbs, 95 calories
- Coors light – 5 carbs, 102 calories
- Michelob ultra-amber – 3.7 carbs, 114 calories
- Natural light – 3.2 carbs, 95 calories
- Miller Lite – 3.2 carbs, 96 calories
- Bud select – 3.1 carbs, 99 calories
- Michelob ultra – 2.6 carbs, 95 calories
- Rolling rock green light = 2.4 carbs, 92 calories
- MGD – 2.4 carbs, 64 calories
- Bud select 55 – 1.9 carbs, 55 calories

You have to watch out, though. Sugar is hidden everywhere. Gin and tonic have 30 grams of carbs. Tonic water has a high sugar content. If your cocktail comes with simple syrup and artificial lime juice, you are probably at 50 grams of sugar. Stay away from popular drinks and mix-ins.

Sweets on the Keto Diet

A lot of people have a sweet tooth and a Keto diet makes just a bit harder to enjoy sweets. But don't worry that doesn't mean there isn't any hope. There are lots of options of sweets you can make yourself. There are even a few store-bought options, but you have to watch out for hidden sugars with those.

The easiest way to satisfy your sweet cravings is to make your own sweets at home. That way you can control what goes into them. While you can find recipes for cakes and pie crusts out there that are Keto-friendly, they often come with a bunch of confusing instructions and expensive ingredients like psyllium husk powder.

I'm going to share with you some delicious sweets that require just a couple of ingredients and no baking time is required. Something as simple as equal parts nut butter and coconut oil melted together, poured into a greased parchment-lined pan, can make a delicious fudge.

Another fun snack is a three-ingredient coconut bar. Melt a cup of coconut oil and mix in three cups of shredded unsweetened coconut flakes. You can mix in some sugar-free sweetener if you would like. Spread this into a parchment lined baking dish and let it set up.

If you like crunch bars, do melt together 1.5 cups sugar-free chocolate chips, 1 cup peanut butter, 0.5 cup monk fruit syrup, and 0.25 cup coconut oil. Once mixed, stir in 1.5 cups of unsweetened shredded coconut and 1.5 cups of nuts or seeds. Pour this into a parchment lined dish and let set up.

One more quick sweet recipe you can make, melt together 2 cups of sugar-free chocolate hazelnut spread, 0.5 cup monk fruit syrup. Mix in 0.75 cup coconut flour. If it is too crumbly add a bit of water to reach a good consistency. Roll the mixture into bite-sized balls. Refrigerate them for 30 minutes.

Keto sweets are really simple. You can go crazy and make fancy cakes and things. You can simply melt together a few things with coconut oil.

Keto-Friendly Snacks

You will likely not experience hunger during the day that prompts you to turn to snacks, but it still doesn't hurt to have some snacks on hand. Snacks are a good thing to have with you when you are taking a trip to keep from having to find something Keto-friendly at a roadside food joint.

Here are ten great snack foods to keep on hand.

1. Macadamia nuts – these have the highest amount of fat and lowest amount of carbs of the nut family.

2. Pecans – these are a great source of magnesium and protein.

3. Beef jerky – this is a great low-carb, high-fat snack and it's convenient. If you don't make your own, make sure you check the packet to see if there are any added sugars.

4. Half an avocado – sprinkle it with some salt and olive oil and you have a great snack.

5. Smoothie with coconut flakes – a quick blend of protein powder, greens, almond milk, and almond butter topped with some coconut flakes is tasty and good.

6. Cheese and meat roll-ups – in a hurry? Roll up some deli meat and cheese for a quick snack.

7. Charcuterie – meat is a perfect option for a snack on Keto.

8. Olives – grab a jar of olives for a high fat snack.

9. String cheese – all types of cheese is fair game for a quick and easy snack on Keto.

10. Hardboiled eggs – it's easy to cook up a few eggs to have on hand if you need a little something to munch on.

Spices, Dressings, and Sauces

Spices, dressings, and sauces are what can sneak in some carbs to your diet. Spices, specifically, can end up your fat burning process. Let's look at some of the best fat burning, low-carb spices that you should have in your pantry.

- Cayenne pepper – the capsaicin in cayenne can up your metabolism for a short time.

- Cinnamon – cinnamon can fight off carb cravings, promote healthier circulation, reduce LDL levels and blood sugar.

- Mustard seed – spicy mustard works like cayenne pepper and can up your metabolism.

- Turmeric – turmeric and minimize fat and lower cholesterol.

- Garlic – this magic spice can control appetite, fight high cholesterol, lower insulin levels, and lower blood sugar.

- Ginger – much like garlic, ginger can fight cholesterol levels and improve metabolism.

- Black pepper – this spice can up your metabolism and help with nutrient absorption.

- Ginseng – studies have found ginseng can help with weight control.

The only spice you really need to watch out for is garlic powder. The rest you could probably not worry about. There's no sense stressing over 0.1 grams of carbs.

Alright, you're good on spices, so your meals are going to have flavor, but what if they're dry. Nobody wants to have a salad without some dressing. There are a lot of Keto recipes out there where you can make your own ketchup, hummus, and creamy salad dressings, but you can buy some of these things too. The most important thing is to read the nutrition label correctly.

The top five condiments you can buy at the store without too much trouble are:

1. Mayonnaise – check to make sure it is made with a healthy fat.

2. Ranch and Caesar dressings – most of the time they won't be made with healthy fats, but they are great options when you're in a pinch, need to get something quick, or are eating out.

3. Butter or ghee – great for a steak topping.

4. Alfredo sauce – check the label to see if you can find a dairy free option.

5. Hot sauce – most don't have any carbs, but do check just to be on the safe side.

Chapter 6: Maintaining

The only way to make sure you stick with any weight loss plan is to make sure that you are prepared and that you keep track of your success.

Start by removing temptations. Go through your house, and get rid of anything that is not Keto-friendly. Now, this can get tricky if you're not the only one living in your house. This is where you need to sit everybody in the house down and let them know what you are doing. Some of them may want to join you. If there are others that aren't partaking, ask them to hide their snacks that you can't have so that you won't see them all the time. If there are refrigerated things that you can't get rid of because they are somebody else's, get solid boxes to store them in so you don't see them.

When you get snacks and foods, pre-portion them so that you can grab and go and not have to worry about using the right amount. It's easy to sit and mindlessly munch on pork rinds—but that's not good. Put your seeds, nuts, pork rinds, sandwich meat, and so on in serving size bags.

Try to aim for your meals to only contain five net carbs. Also, to make sure you stick to your plan, keep a good journal. Track what you eat and how you exercise—and your moods will help keep you on target.

The important thing is to make a commitment to yourself that you are going to stick with for a certain number of days. At the end of those days, you will reevaluate, create a new goal, and reward yourself. You shouldn't write a timeframe that is an infinite amount of time. It's easier to stick to something if you make your goals small and manageable.

Setting Goals

When you are setting your goals, you want to make sure that they are SMART goals. These are goals that you can feasibly move forward with and start seeing results. The point of your goals is for you to be able to be working towards something that is actually attainable. Using the criteria that I'm going to give you, decide on the things you want to change the most through your Keto diet. Will it fit into the SMART structure? If it does, then you can officially set your goal and start tracking your results.

- S – specific: would anybody that has basic knowledge of the subject be able to understand it?

- M – measurable: are you able to tell how far away you are from reaching it, and will you know when you have obtained it?

- A – achievable: will you be able to eventually reach the goal?

- R – realistic: with your time, resources, and knowledge, will you be able to reach your goal?

- T – trackable: is there an accurate way to track your progress?

Tracking Results

Now you have to figure out how you are going to keep track of your results. You can put in all of your efforts, but if you don't know where you're going and how close you are, it will get confusing and frustrating.

The way you track your goals will depend on what your health goal is. Take a moment to think about the best ways you can measure your progress. How are you going to be able to best see the changes happen not just day-to-day but month-to-month and so on?

The following are some good ways to track progress based on goals.

When your goal is weight loss:

- Take a picture before you start and then take a new picture every month to compare.

- You can do a hydrostatic body-fast test at regular times.

- You can weigh yourself, but make sure that you don't become a slave to the scale. Your body weight will fluctuate daily, and other things like body composition, are better indicators.

- Use a urine test for Ketone levels every day to make sure that you stay in Ketosis.

- Measure yourself. Do measurements of your chest, neck, waist, hips, thighs, and arms before, and then measure yourself again at regular intervals.

When your goal is to improve your mental state:

- Keep a daily journal about how you mentally feel. You can rate your clarity on a scale of one to ten and then explain why you feel that way.

- Track your productivity at work. Write down how much you were able to accomplish, how many projects got finished, or the number of breaks you had to take.

When your goal is better physical performance:

- Keep a daily journal and write down how you feel physically and when you work out. You can also rate your energy level from one to ten before you work out and after.

- Write down the specific results you had at the gym, like distance ran, weight lifted, or the number of reps.

- Keep up with what you ate before and after your workout. Along with your gym results, write down when you ate around your workout schedule.

It's important that you track often. You could feel discouraged from time to time, but if you keep track of your progress, it can keep you motivated. Remember, it's perfectly okay if things don't work out exactly as planned.

Chapter 7: Weight Loss Guide Routine

To help you get started on your journey towards a Keto diet, here is a 30-day meal plan that will help kick-start your diet.

Day 1

Breakfast: Two fried eggs – 1-gram net carb

Lunch: 1/3 cup of hummus with pork rinds – 9 grams of net carb

Dinner: Chicken salad with balsamic vinegar dressing – 6 grams of net carb

Day 2

Breakfast: Two eggs and two slices of bacon – 1-gram net carb

Lunch: An avocado with pork rinds – 2 grams of net carb

Dinner: Tuna salad with two hard boil eggs, bibb lettuce, a half cup of almonds, an apple, and a cucumber – 13 grams of net carb

Day 3

Breakfast: Bulletproof coffee – 0-gram net carb

Lunch: Serving of sunflower seeds – 4 grams of net carbs

Dinner: Two ounces of turkey breast, hard boil egg, a quarter cup of cherry tomatoes, an ounce of sharp cheddar, four pita bites, two tablespoons almonds – 13 grams of net carbs

Day 4

Breakfast: One boiled egg with a tablespoon mayo – 1-gram net carb

Lunch: 1/3 cup of hummus with pork rinds – 9 grams of net carb

Dinner: Chicken salad with balsamic vinegar dressing – 6 grams of net carb

Day 5

Breakfast: Romaine lettuce leaf with a half-ounce of butter, an ounce of cheese, half an avocado, and a cherry tomato – 3 grams of net carb

Lunch: String cheese – 1 gram of net carb

Dinner: Tuna salad with two hard boil eggs, bibb lettuce, a half cup of almonds, an apple, and a cucumber – 13 grams of net carb

Day 6

Breakfast: An avocado with three ounces of deli turkey, an ounce of lettuce, and an ounce and a half of cream cheese – 9 grams of net carb

Lunch: Serving of pork rinds – 0 grams of net carb

Dinner: Chicken salad with balsamic vinegar dressing – 6 grams of net carb

Day 7

Breakfast: Two eggs and two slices of bacon – 1-gram net carb

Lunch: An avocado with pork rinds – 2 grams of net carb

Dinner: Tuna salad with two hard boil eggs, bibb lettuce, a half cup of almonds, an apple, and a cucumber – 13 grams of net carb

Day 8

Breakfast: Two fried eggs – 1-gram net carb

Lunch: 1/3 cup of hummus with pork rinds – 9 grams of net carb

Dinner: Chicken salad with balsamic vinegar dressing – 6 grams of net carb

Day 9

Breakfast: A cup of coffee with four tablespoons heavy cream – 2 grams of net carb

Lunch: An avocado with pork rinds – 2 grams of net carb

Dinner: Two ounces of turkey breast, hard boil egg, a quarter cup of cherry tomatoes, an ounce of sharp cheddar, four pita bites, two tablespoons almonds – 13 grams of net carbs

Day 10

Breakfast: Two hardboiled eggs mashed into three ounces of butter – 1-gram net carb

Lunch: Quest bar – 5 grams of net carb

Dinner: Roll three slices of cheese in three slices of turkey and serve with half of an avocado, cucumber slices, blueberries, and almonds – 13 grams of net carb

Day 11

Breakfast: An avocado with three ounces of deli turkey, an ounce of lettuce, and an ounce and a half of cream cheese – 9 grams of net carb

Lunch: Serving of pork rinds – 0 grams of net carb

Dinner: Chicken salad with balsamic vinegar dressing – 6 grams of net carb

Day 12

Breakfast: An avocado fill with a third of a cup of mayo and three ounces of smoked salmon – 6 grams of net carb

Lunch: Full-fat laughing cow cheese – 1-gram net carb

Dinner: Roll three slices of cheese in three slices of turkey and serve with half of an avocado, cucumber slices, blueberries, and almonds – 13 grams of net carb

Day 13

Breakfast: Two scrambled eggs – 1-gram net carb

Lunch: 1/3 cup of hummus with pork rinds – 9 grams of net carb

Dinner: Chicken salad with balsamic vinegar dressing – 6 grams of net carb

Day 14

Breakfast: Romaine lettuce leaf with a half-ounce of butter, an ounce of cheese, half an avocado, and a cherry tomato – 3 grams of net carb

Lunch: String cheese – 1 gram of net carb

Dinner: Two ounces of turkey breast, hard boil egg, a quarter cup of cherry tomatoes, an ounce of sharp cheddar, four pita bites, two tablespoons almonds – 13 grams of net carbs

Day 15

Breakfast: A cup of coffee with four tablespoons heavy cream – 2 grams of net carb

Lunch: An avocado with pork rinds – 2 grams of net carb

Dinner: Tuna salad with two hard boil eggs, bibb lettuce, a half cup of almonds, an apple, and a cucumber – 13 grams of net carb

Day 16

Breakfast: One boiled eggs with a tablespoon mayo – 1-gram net carb

Lunch: 1/3 cup of hummus with pork rinds – 9 grams of net carb

Dinner: Chicken salad with balsamic vinegar dressing – 6 grams of net carb

Day 17

Breakfast: An avocado with three ounces of deli turkey, an ounce of lettuce, and an ounce and a half of cream cheese – 9 grams of net carb

Lunch: Serving of pork rinds – 0 grams of net carb

Dinner: Roll three slices of cheese in three slices of turkey and serve with half of an avocado, cucumber slices, blueberries, and almonds – 13 grams of net carb

Day 18

Breakfast: Bulletproof coffee – 0-gram net carb

Lunch: Serving of sunflower seeds – 4 grams of net carbs

Dinner: Two ounces of turkey breast, hard boil egg, a quarter cup of cherry tomatoes, an ounce of sharp cheddar, four pita bites, two tablespoons almonds – 13 grams of net carbs

Day 19

Breakfast: Two hardboiled eggs mashed into three ounces of butter – 1-gram net carb

Lunch: An avocado with pork rinds – 2 grams of net carb

Dinner: Tuna salad with two hard boil eggs, bibb lettuce, a half cup of almonds, an apple, and a cucumber – 13 grams of net carb

Day 20

Breakfast: Two fried eggs – 1-gram net carb

Lunch: 1/3 cup of hummus with pork rinds – 9 grams of net carb

Dinner: Chicken salad with balsamic vinegar dressing – 6 grams of net carb

Day 21

Breakfast: Two eggs and two slices of bacon – 1-gram net carb

Lunch: Quest bar – 5 grams of net carb

Dinner: Two ounces of turkey breast, hard boil egg, a quarter cup of cherry tomatoes, an ounce of sharp cheddar, four pita bites, two tablespoons almonds – 13 grams of net carbs

Day 22

Breakfast: A cup of coffee with four tablespoons heavy cream – 2 grams of net carb

Lunch: An avocado with pork rinds – 2 grams of net carb

Dinner: Tuna salad with two hard boil eggs, bibb lettuce, a half cup of almonds, an apple, and a cucumber – 13 grams of net carb

Day 23

Breakfast: An avocado fill with a third of a cup of mayo and three ounces of smoked salmon – 6 grams of net carb

Lunch: Full-fat laughing cow cheese – 1-gram net carb

Dinner: Roll three slices of cheese in three slices of turkey and serve with half of an avocado, cucumber slices, blueberries, and almonds – 13 grams of net carb

Day 24

Breakfast: An avocado with three ounces of deli turkey, an ounce of lettuce, and an ounce and a half of cream cheese – 9 grams of net carb

Lunch: Serving of pork rinds – 0 grams of net carb

Dinner: Chicken salad with balsamic vinegar dressing – 6 grams of net carb

Day 25

Breakfast: Two hardboiled eggs mashed into three ounces of butter – 1-gram net carb

Lunch: Quest bar – 5 grams of net carb

Dinner: Two ounces of turkey breast, hard boil egg, a quarter cup of cherry tomatoes, an ounce of sharp cheddar, four pita bites, two tablespoons almonds – 13 grams of net carbs

Day 26

Breakfast: Two fried eggs – 1-gram net carb

Lunch: 1/3 cup of hummus with pork rinds – 9 grams of net carb

Dinner: Chicken salad with balsamic vinegar dressing – 6 grams of net carb

Day 27

Breakfast: Two scrambled eggs with an avocado and two ounces of smoked salmon – 5 grams of net carb

Lunch: Full-fat laughing cow cheese – 1-gram net carb

Dinner: Tuna salad with two hard boil eggs, bibb lettuce, a half cup of almonds, an apple, and a cucumber – 13 grams of net carb

Day 28

Breakfast: Two scrambled eggs – 1-gram net carb

Lunch: 1/3 cup of hummus with pork rinds – 9 grams of net carb

Dinner: Chicken salad with balsamic vinegar dressing – 6 grams of net carb

Day 29

Breakfast: Romaine lettuce leaf with a half-ounce of butter, an ounce of cheese, half an avocado, and a cherry tomato – 3 grams of net carb

Lunch: String cheese – 1 gram of net carb

Dinner: Two ounces of turkey breast, hard boil egg, a quarter cup of cherry tomatoes, an ounce of sharp cheddar, four pita bites, two tablespoons almonds – 13 grams of net carbs

Day 30

Breakfast: One boiled egg with a tablespoon mayo – 1-gram net carb

Lunch: 1/3 cup of hummus with pork rinds – 9 grams of net carb

Dinner: Chicken salad with balsamic vinegar dressing – 6 grams of net carb

Chapter 8: Ten Most Popular and Tastiest Recipes

Asian Beef Salad

What you will need:

- Ribeye steaks, 2/3 pound
- Chili flakes, 1 teaspoon
- Grated ginger, 1 tablespoon
- Fish sauce, 1 tablespoon
- Olive oil, 1 tablespoon

Salad:

- Sesame seeds, 1 tablespoon
- Cilantro
- Red onion, .5
- Lettuce, 3 ounces
- Cucumber, 2 ounces
- Cherry tomatoes, 3 ounces
- Scallions, 2

Mayo:

- Pepper
- Salt
- Lime juice, .5 tablespoon
- Sesame oil, 1 tablespoon
- Olive oil, .5 c
- Dijon mustard, 1 teaspoon
- Egg yolk

What you will do:

1. Start by mixing the mustard and egg yolk together. As you whisk, slowly add in the olive oil. This can be done either with an immersion blender or by hand. Once the mayonnaise has become emulsified, add in the sesame oil, spices, and lime juice. Set the mayo to the side.

2. Mix together the olive oil, chili flakes, ginger, and fish sauce—and then add the mixture to a plastic bag. Add the ribeye in and let it marinate together for 15 minutes.

3. Chop up all of the ingredients for the salad, minus the scallions. Split them between two plates.

4. Heat a skillet and add the sesame seeds and allow them to dry roast for a few minutes. Place them to the side.

5. Pat the meat off and fry in the skillet for a few minutes and each side. Cook to your desired doneness, but with this dish, it's best cooked to medium.

6. Fry the scallions for a bit in the skillet.

7. Cut the steak into thin slices. Add the scallions and beef to the top of the vegetables and top with the sesame seeds. Serve with the mayo.

- 7 grams – net carb
- 98 grams – fat
- 34 grams – protein
- 2 servings

Breakfast Sandwich

What you will need:

- Tabasco
- Pepper
- Salt
- Cheddar cheese slices, 2 ounce
- Smoked deli ham, 1 ounce
- Eggs, 4
- Butter, 2 tablespoons

What you will do:

1. Place the butter in a skillet. Fry each of the eggs in the skillet until done to your liking. Make sure you pepper and salt them.

2. The fried eggs are the bread to your sandwich. Add the deli ham and cheese, and then top with a second egg. Sprinkle them with some Tabasco sauce if you want.

- 2 grams – net carb
- 30 grams – fat
- 20 grams – protein
- 2 servings

Meat Pie

What you will need:

- Water, .5 c
- Tomato paste, 4 tablespoons
- Dried oregano, 1 tablespoon
- Pepper
- Salt
- Ground beef, 20 ounces
- Butter, 2 tablespoons
- Chopped garlic clove
- Chopped onion, .5

Crust:

- Water, 4 tablespoons
- Egg
- Olive oil, 3 tablespoons
- Pinch salt
- Baking powder, 1 teaspoon
- Ground psyllium husk powder, 1 tablespoon
- Coconut flour, 4 tablespoons
- Sesame seeds, 4 tablespoons
- Almond flour, .75 c

Topping:

- Shredded cheese, 7 ounces
- Cottage cheese, 8 ounces

What you will do:

1. Start by setting your oven to 350. Add the butter to a skillet and cook the garlic and onion until the onion becomes soft. Add in the beef and cook until browned. Mix in the pepper, oregano, basil, and salt.

2. Mix in the tomato paste and water. Turn the heat down and let it simmer for 20 minutes. As this is cooking, take the time to make the crust.

3. Place all of the dough ingredients in a food processor and combine until it forms a ball. This can also be done by hand if you don't have a processor.

4. Grease a springform pan and lay a piece of parchment paper in the bottom. Spread the dough onto the bottom up to the sides with greased fingers. Let this bake for 10 to 15 minutes. Pour the meat mixture into the baked crust.

5. Mix together the topping ingredients and spread them across the meat. Allow the pie to bake for 30 to 40 minutes, or until it becomes golden.

- 7 grams – net carb
- 47 grams – fat
- 38 grams – protein
- 6 servings

Western Omelet

What you will need:

- Diced deli ham, 5 ounces
- Chopped bell pepper, .5
- Chopped onion, .5
- Butter, 2 ounces
- Shredded cheese, 3 ounces
- Pepper
- Salt
- Heavy whipping cream, 2 tablespoons
- Eggs, 6

What you will do:

6. Beat together the eggs, heavy cream, pepper, and salt until frothy. Mix in half of the shredded cheese.

7. Add the butter to a skillet and cook the ham, peppers, and onion. Pour in the egg mixture and cook until almost firm.

8. Turn the heat down and top with the remaining cheese. Fold in half and enjoy.

- 6 grams – net carb
- 58 grams – fat
- 40 grams – protein
- 2 servings

Avocado Hummus

What you will need:

- Pepper, .25 teaspoon
- Salt, .5 teaspoon
- Cumin, .5 teaspoon
- Pressed garlic
- Lemon juice, .5
- Tahini, .25 c
- Sunflower seeds, .25 c
- Olive oil, .5 c
- Cilantro, .5 c
- Avocados, 3

What you will do:

1. Halve the avocados, take out the pits, and spoon out the flesh. Place everything in a blender and mix until completely smooth. Add water, lemon juice, or oil if you need to loosen the mixture bit.

- 4 grams – net carb
- 41 grams – fat
- 5 grams – protein
- 6 servings

Cheeseburger

What you will need:

- Butter, 2 ounces – frying
- Chopped oregano, 2 tablespoons
- Paprika, 2 teaspoons
- Onion powder, 2 teaspoons
- Garlic powder, 2 teaspoons
- Shredded cheese, 7 ounces
- Ground beef, 25 ounces

Salsa:

- Cilantro
- Salt
- Olive oil, 1 tablespoon
- Avocado
- Scallions, 2
- Tomatoes, 2

Toppings:

- Pickled jalapenos, .25 c
- Lettuce, 5 ounces
- Sliced pickles, .5 c
- Dijon mustard, 4 tablespoons
- Cooked bacon, 5 ounces
- Mayonnaise, .75 c

What you will do:

1. Chop all of the ingredients up for the salsa and mix them together. Set to the side.

2. Combine the beef with half the cheese and the all the seasonings. Form into four burgers and cook however you would prefer. Top the burgers with the remaining cheese when they are almost done.

3. Serve the burgers with lettuce, pickle, and mustard. Top with the salsa.

- 8 grams – net carb
- 104 grams – fat
- 54 grams – protein
- 4 servings

Coconut Porridge

What you will need:

- Pinch salt
- Coconut cream, 4 tablespoon
- Pinch ground psyllium husk powder
- Coconut flour, 1 tablespoon
- Egg
- Butter, 1 ounce

What you will do:

4. Place all of your ingredients in a pot. Mix everything together and let it heat over low. Stir this constantly until it reaches your desired texture. Serve this with some coconut milk and berries if you want.

- 4 grams – net carb
- 49 grams – fat
- 9 grams – protein

Bake Brie Cheese

What you will need:

- Pepper
- Salt
- Olive oil, 1 tablespoon
- Rosemary, 1 tablespoon
- Garlic clove
- Pecans, 2 ounces
- Brie Cheese, 9 ounces

What you will do:

1. Set your oven to 400. Lay the cheese on a parchment lined baking sheet.

2. Mince up the herbs and garlic, and chop the nuts. Combine them together with the olive oil. Add in some pepper and salt. Pour this over the cheese and let it bake for ten minutes.

- 1 gram – net carb
- 31 grams – fat
- 14 grams – protein
- 4 servings

Hamburger in Tomato Sauce

What you will need:

Patties:

- Butter, .25 teaspoon
- Olive oil, 1 tablespoon
- Chopped parsley, 2 ounces
- Pepper, .25 teaspoon
- Salt, 1 teaspoon
- Crumbled feta, 3 ounces
- Egg
- Ground beef, 25 ounces

Gravy:

- Pepper
- Salt
- Tomato paste, 2 tablespoons
- Chopped parsley, 1 ounce
- Heavy whipping cream, .75 c

Fried Cabbage:

- Pepper
- Salt
- Butter, 4.25 ounces
- Shredded cabbage, 25 ounces

What you will do:

1. Blend all of the patty ingredients together. Form the mixture into eight patties. Place the oil and butter in a skillet and cook for ten minutes, or until cooked through. Flip them a couple of times while cooking.

2. When almost done, add the whipping cream and tomato paste to the pan. Stir and allow it to simmer for a couple of

minutes. Season with some pepper and salt. Sprinkle everything with parsley before serving.

3. For the cabbage: add the butter to a skillet and fry the cabbage for 15 minutes, or until wilted and browned on the edges. Season with some pepper and salt.

4. Serve the patties with the cabbage.

- 10 grams – net carb
- 78 grams – fat
- 43 grams – protein
- 4 servings

Roast Beef

What you will need:

- Pepper
- Salt
- Olive oil, 2 tablespoons
- Lettuce, 2 ounces
- Dijon mustard, 1 tablespoon
- Mayonnaise, 5 c
- Scallion
- Radishes, 6
- Avocado
- Cheddar cheese, 5 ounces
- Deli roast beef, 7 ounces

What you will do:

5. Lay the radishes, avocado, cheese, and roast beef on two plates. Add on the mustard, onion, and mayonnaise. Serve with some lettuce and drizzle with some olive oil.

- 6 grams – net carb
- 98 grams – fat
- 38 grams – protein
- 2 servings

Chapter 9: Diseases Treated by Keto

The Ketogenic diet has an interesting effect on many different diseases. In this chapter, we are going to quickly look over some of the big diseases that a Keto diet can help combat.

Cancer

The Ketogenic diet is able to starve cancer cells. Otto Warburg, a leading cell biologist, found that cancer cells weren't able to flourish with energy created through cellular respiration but instead needed glucose fermentation. Other cancer researchers, including Dr. Thomas Seyfried, agree and have found that cancer cells can also be fueled from the fermentation of glutamine.

With a Ketogenic diet, you lower carb intake, and it reduces the levels of glucose, which will feed cancer cells. Once your body reaches Ketosis, it will help in depleting the energy supply of cancer cells.

Cancer cells vary from normal cells in many different ways, but one of their traits that is the most interesting regards insulin receptors. On their cellular surface, they have ten times more insulin receptors. This allows cancer cells to fill their self on glucose and nutrients that come from the bloodstream very quickly. As you consume more glucose as your main source of energy, cancer cells are going to continue to spread and thrive. It isn't surprising that the lowest odds of survival in cancer patients are among those that have higher blood sugar levels.

The mitochondria in the cancer cells are damaged—and it lacks the ability to create energy through aerobic respiration. They aren't able to metabolize fatty acids to use for energy. This is the reason why cancer cells thrive in environments that are oxygen-depleted. Instead, cancer cells are able to metabolize amino acids and glucose. Restricting the amino acid glutamine or glucose is important for starving cancer.

Crohn's Disease

Almost every child and adult will experience stomach issues at one time or another, but millions suffer from autoimmune problems like Crohn's disease. These types of digestive diseases, which don't have a medical cure, will require lifetime care for the sufferer.

A Ketogenic diet is able to improve symptoms of Crohn's disease by getting rid of inflammatory foods and gut irritants, like:

- Some high fiber veggies and fruits.
- Dairy
- Refined and processed foods
- Legumes and beans
- Pseudo grains that include buckwheat, quinoa, and amaranth
- Grains like rice, corn, oats, barley, rye, and wheat

With inflammation being reduced, the gastrointestinal system will start to heal. After it has been healed, some people can re-introduce foods that used to trigger their symptoms, like fibrous fruits and veggies, seeds, and nuts.

Diabetes

Duke University Medical Center was one of the first to start investigating how a Ketogenic diet impacts diabetes. They recruited 28 overweight participants who had type 2 diabetes and underwent a 16-week intervention trial.

They had a mean BMI of 42.2 and a mean age of 56. They were all either Caucasian or African American. They consumed a Ketogenic diet where they had to eat less than 20 grams of net carbs each day while they reduced their diabetes medication.

Of the 21 subjects who successfully completed the intervention, the researchers found that they had a 16% decrease in hemoglobin A1c from their baseline. They had an average decrease on 19.2 pounds and their average blood glucose levels went down by 16.6%. In the end, the majority of subjects were able to reduce or discontinue their diabetes medications.

Most studies look at the effects of the Keto diet on type 2 diabetes, but it is still a viable treatment for type 1. There aren't any formal studies examining how the Keto diet affects type 1 diabetics. A study from 2012 did look at the effects of reduced carb diets on type 1 diabetes patients.

In this study, researchers studied 48 subjects with a mean age of 24. For the ones who stuck to the diet, their hemoglobin A1c reduced from 7.7% to 6.4%.

Acne and Skin Problems

Italian researchers, in 2012, published an article that looked at the possible benefits that a Keto diet could have for acne and skin problems. They found that skin problem could be treated in three ways through a Keto diet:

1. It reduces insulin levels. A Keto diet can dramatically reduce insulin levels.

2. By reducing inflammation. Inflammation is the reason why acne becomes so tender, red, and sore.

3. By decreasing IGF-1 levels. The reduction of IGF-1 levels helps regulate sebum production, which can prevent pores from getting clogged.

Depression and Anxiety

You will constantly find stories of how a Ketogenic diet has helped people fight off depression and anxiety. According to Jennifer Wider, MD, says that a Keto diet could cause certain bodily processes that could fight off depression.

Your body produces more GABA, which a major neurotransmitter, while on a Keto diet. When GABA levels are low, you are more likely to experience depression and anxiety. When they are high, it helps stave off these problems.

Weight loss is also able to help relieve symptoms of mental illnesses, especially if one's depression is linked to being overweight.

Alzheimer's Disease

We've always believed that there was no way to reverse Alzheimer's disease, but a Keto diet may be able to help slow down the progress. The brain is an energy hog and demands a constant fuel supply. When a person has dementia, their brain has a hard time burning glucose, which causes sluggish brain activity, brain shrinkage, and death of brain cells.

People with Alzheimer's have an energy crisis on their hands. Luckily, except when Alzheimer's has advanced, the brain does great at burning Ketones.

In one study that placed participants with mild to moderate Alzheimer's on a Keto diet for four months, and had them track the urine Ketones each morning. They had to perform cognitive tests at the beginning, after three months, and then four months later after they had started following their old diet again.

Ten of 15 participants were able to successfully and safely complete the study. The ten that finished had mild Alzheimer's. Those with moderate were not able to finish the study due to caregiver burden.

The cognitive test results in those ten people improved significantly for nine of them. The improvements in their tests disappeared after they returned to their regular diets.

Inflammation and Chronic Pain

Opiates are the most powerful drugs that are used to treat pain, but they pose serious problems and can be addictive. A Ketogenic diet can alleviate pain because of several of its biochemical consequences.

These include the activation of peroxisome proliferator-activated receptors, increased adenosine, decreased neural activity, and decreased reactive oxygen species. Through all of this, a Keto diet can reduce inflammatory and neuropathic pain. Unfortunately, there aren't any actual human or animal tests on the efficacy.

Pregnancy

A big question some women have is if they can follow a Ketogenic diet while pregnant. A lot of people worry that their carb intake will be too low, but there's no real evidence that eating real foods on a Keto diet will harm a fetus.

A lean human body is 74% fat and 26% protein by calories. The human cell's structure is made up of fat and is the preferred fuel source for mitochondria. A fetus will naturally use Ketones before and right after birth.

In the later stages of a pregnancy, there is a greater breakdown of fat deposits, which plays a large part in fetal development. The fetus is able to use transported placental fatty acids, glycerol, and Ketone bodies.

Greater Ketogenesis in a fasted state or with MCT oils will create an easy transference of Ketones to the baby which will let the maternal Ketone bodies reach the baby. Once there, the Ketones are able to be used as fuel for oxidative metabolism.

While pregnant, women will often become more sensitive to carbs because of an evolutionary adaption where they become a bit insulin resistant to allow a good flow of nutrients to travel to the developing fetus.

Breast milk is higher in fat than formula, which is full of sugar and carbs. This means if a baby is breastfed, they will likely be in a Ketosis state most of the time. That makes them Keto-adapted. Ketosis can help a baby's brain develop. This means that it is okay to follow a Ketogenic diet while pregnant.

Chapter 10: Myths and Common Questions

There is a lot of false information surrounding the Ketogenic diet—so much, that many people are afraid to try it. We are going to talk about a few of the most popular myths.

You are only going to lose weight following a Keto diet.

This diet will help people lose weight and burn fat. If you don't want to lose weight, you can still follow the diet to maintain your weight or to help you gain some weight.

Could you really gain weight on this diet? It's possible, if you don't do the diet the right way and never get into Ketosis.

There is a lot of controversy about the low-carb, high-fat diet because some people think you lose weight because of the low-calorie intake. Others think it is because of hormonal changes the diet causes. Many experts agree that it doesn't matter what type of diet somebody does—if your calorie intake exceeds your needs or activity level, you will gain weight instead of losing weight.

If you are eating more calories than you need, even if they come from protein and healthy fats, you will see the number on your scale increase.

If you are not looking to lose weight, should you still do a Keto diet? There are many benefits of the Keto diet that go far beyond weight loss. This diet can help your body normalize blood sugar, regulate hormone production, improve digestive health, improve cognitive function, and possibly reduce the risk of getting heart disease or diabetes.

There's no science to back up the Keto diet.

If you've have paid attention so far, there have been many case studies done looking at the effects of a Ketogenic diet. Specifically, there have been studies done looking at its effects on obesity, cancer, muscle loss, insulin resistance, Alzheimer's disease, type 2 diabetes, dyslipidemia, epilepsy, and high blood pressure.

You lose muscle mass.

The Keto diet can help you gain muscle mass if done correctly. The AHA has claimed that a low-carb diet can cause a person to lose muscle tissue. There are no physiological requirements for your body to have carbs, and as long as you don't let your protein intake slack, you shouldn't lose muscle mass. Your protein intake is what protects your muscles, not carbs.

Exercising is out of the question.

Exercising can help everybody, including ones doing a Keto diet. You might not feel as energized when the body is transitioning into Ketosis but this will lessen as your body adjusts. Even during high-intensity workouts, won't cause your performance to decline.

You do not need to stop working out while on the Keto diet. You might have to modify your workouts a bit. If you can handle it, exercising while in Ketosis will burn fat two to three times faster. It can also maintain blood glucose levels and you will notice less fatigue with activity.

To make sure you help your body during workouts, you need to eat enough calories including those from fat. Make sure you let your body recover between tough workouts.

If you find yourself struggling very bad while working out and having a hard time recovering, then try eating more carbs just before exercising. If you fast while on the Keto diet, save your high-intensity workout for times when you are more fueled up.

Everybody will suffer from the Keto flu.

Everybody is going to react differently when their body adapts to Ketosis. This makes it hard to figure what a person is going to experience, how severe their reactions are going to be, and how long it will last. Some transition more smoothly than others. Some may experience fatigue, brain fog, sleep problems, and digestive problems for the week after they reach Ketosis. Keep in mind, these are only temporary problems and will go away with time, with more water, or with more salt.

You can eat all types of fat as people do on Atkin's.

Even though the majority of your calories should come from fat, this doesn't mean you should consume all the saturated fats that you want. Keto diet wants you to eat healthy fats, whereas the Atkin's diet allows all types of fatty foods. A lot of people who follow a Keto diet will stay away from processed meats like bacon, sausage, and salami.

You also have the option of eating clean on Keto and avoiding cheeses, bad quality meats, trans fats, fast food, fried foods, and processed foods. Most people who follow a Keto diet will turn towards healthier options like EVOO, coconut oil, grass-fed butter and meats, nuts, avocados, wild caught fish, pasture-raised poultry, and organic eggs.

Keto is dangerous.

As with anything in life, there are downsides to a Keto diet, but it's not dangerous. Most bad things like kidney stones, increased risk of heart disease, vitamin and mineral deficiencies, high cholesterol, decreased bone density, and gastrointestinal distress can be reduced with water and supplements.

As long you as you make sure you are getting plenty of electrolytes and water, you shouldn't have a problem.

10 Important Questions

Now that we have gotten the myths out of the way, let's look at the ten most popular questions concerning the Ketogenic diet.

1. How soon will I hit Ketosis?

   You have to allow your body enough time to adjust to the diet. This means you have to be strict with your carb intake. If you can't remain consistent, then you may not ever reach Ketosis. That said, if you stay consistent, reaching Ketosis can take anywhere from two to seven days. It will all depend on the foods you eat, your body type, and activity level.

2. Do I need to count calories?

   Yes, calories do matter. Calories are what will affect if you lose weight or not, so you do need to eat in a deficit of calories in versus calories out. But, with a Keto diet, calories don't tend to be as much of a concern. Fats and protein will make up most of your diet, and it will take fewer calories to make you feel full than with a diet high in carbs.

3. Can I eat too much fat?

   Yes, you could end up eating too much fat. This goes back to the calories. You have to make sure you keep your calories in a deficit, so it is possible to consume too many calories from fat. This is why you should keep a macro and calorie tracker on your phone so that you can put in the foods that you eat. You will be less likely to over-consume that way.

4. Should I take supplements?

It's not a bad idea to start taking supplements since you will be cutting out food sources that would naturally provide with these vitamins and minerals. Start taking them especially if you start to feel crampy or just unusual once you start your diet. The following supplements can help you:

- Potassium
- Vitamin D
- Vitamin B complex
- Magnesium
- Multivitamin for men
- Multivitamin for women

Make sure that you talk to your doctor first if you are on any other medications because there could be an interaction.

5. Should I worry if I exercise?

No. Exercising is completely safe on a Keto diet, as we discussed earlier. But a Keto diet can affect the way you exercise. If you do a lot of cardio work like running, biking, dancing, and so on, then you can get away with a little more carbs. If you like to lift weights, then you may have to adjust your goals. Carbs do help with muscle performance and recovery. That's why a lot of strength trainers will follow a cyclical or targeted Ketogenic diet, meaning the up their carb intake right before a weight session. You don't have to do this, though. You may just have to lower your weight the number of reps and sets you perform.

6. I've stalled in my weight loss, what now?

Everybody will probably hit a plateau on any diet. There are a lot of things that could cause this, but there are just as many things to help you work through it. Here are a few suggestions:

- Switch to measuring yourself instead of weighing

- Cut out processed food.
- Check food labels for hidden carbs.
- Cut out some artificial sweeteners.
- Cut out nuts.
- Lower your carb intake.
- Increase your fat intake.
- Quit eating dairy.

7. I'm constipated, what should I do?

It's not uncommon for people who start a Keto diet to have irregular bowel movements. The following list is a few things that you can do to fix you bowel problems:

- Add a magnesium supplement
- Up your water consumption
- Drink coffee or tea
- Eat chia or flax seeds
- Consume more veggies that have high fiber content
- If you eat a lot of nuts, quit
- Try consuming a tablespoon of coconut oil

8. What do I do if I feel crampy?

Headaches and brain fog is a common issue for people who are just starting a Keto diet. Since you will urinate a lot more, you will lose a lot of water. Add that to all the fat burning that will be happening, and you have a recipe for disaster. Urinating more will cause a loss of electrolytes and you have to replace these. Add more salt and water to your diet to combat this problem.

9. How can I tell if I'm in Ketosis?

A lot of people will use *Ketostix* to figure out if they are in Ketosis. These are available online and in most pharmacies, but they aren't completely accurate. You will urinate on them each morning and if they turn purple or pink, you are producing enough Ketones. If it comes out darker than that, then you are probably dehydrated and you Ketone levels are really concentrated.

10. Am I going to lose a lot of weight?

How much weight you lose will depend on you. Exercising can help you lose more. If you completely cut out wheat products, dairy, and artificial sweeteners, you will probably lose more. Just know that first big drop in weight that you will experience after a week or two is mainly water weight. You probably haven't burned that much fat yet. Ketosis has a diuretic effect on the body. The next drop will be fat as long as you have remained in Ketosis.

Chapter 11: Popular Keto Celebrities and Athletes

Vanessa Hudgens

Vanessa Hudgens has taken charge of her career and her diet—and through the Keto diet, she's gotten the best shape of her life. The star has removed refined sugars, dairy, and carbs from her diet. Since she started the Ketogenic diet, Vanessa has dropped ten pounds.

The key to her success was avocados. She made sure to eat one per day. She explained, "If I'm not getting enough, my body holds on to calories. We've been trained to think that fats are bad, but they're so good."

She adds Soul Cycling to her routine as well. When she worked to drop the 20 pounds she had to put on for her movie *Gimme Shelter*, she liked grabbing a front-row seat. This gave her the motivation to pedal faster. She makes sure to grab a class when she can, and she also does circuit training and Pilates.

Vanessa starts her down out with half an avocado, bacon, and eggs—and as the day progresses, she balances her healthy fats and protein with lots of produce. She normally has a salad with dark meat chicken for lunch with a half of an avocado. For dinner, she usually has a grilled steak or salmon with sautéed veggies.

She also tops her diet with some detox teas. She specifically uses Flat Tummy Tea for 28 days to help combat bloating. She rounds out her healthy Ketogenic diet with yoga. Yoga is what helps her center herself after she films an intense movie.

LeBron James and Ray Allen

LeBron adopted a Ketogenic-style Paleo diet a few years back, eliminated nearly all carbs, sugar, and dairy. He followed the strict diet for 67 and said he did so to test his "mental fortitude" and his willpower. During this time, his diet consisted of low-sugar fruits, vegetables, fish, and meat.

For lunch, he liked to have salads. He shared a couple of his meals on Instagram. One was an arugula salad topped with cashews, mangoes, strawberries, and chicken, with a light vinaigrette. Another one of his meals with lobster salad and mango chutney.

LeBron has never come out and said how much weight he lost exactly, but Brain Windhorst, an ESPN reporter who has a lot of access to James, estimated his weight loss to be anywhere from 12 to 20 pounds.

The 6'8" basketball star weighed around 270 the season prior to his Keto diet. The following season, he was down to 250. LeBron had been inspired by the transformation of his former Miami Heat teammate, Ray Allen. Ray had gotten super-fit when he switched to a low-carb Paleo diet during the summer of 2013.

Allen had come back after the summer break a lot better shape than he had been the year before after he adopted his sugar-free, low-carb Paleo diet. Allen didn't start the diet for weight loss. He said that his new diet provided him with more stamina and improves is workout recovery. He also motivated Dwayne Wade.

Ohio State University professor and dietitian, Dr. Jeff Volek, said James' weight loss was because of his Ketogenic-inspired eating plan. Volek explained that many athletes have started to favor high-fat, low-carb diets to lose weight fast and change how their fat composition.

Halle Berry

At 51, Halle Berry looks amazing and does that with the help of a Ketogenic diet and great genetics. She follows a Keto diet for weight management and to manage her diabetes, which she was diagnosed with at 22.

Following the very low-carb, moderate-protein, and high-fat encourages her to burn fats instead of carbs for energy. Halle fills up on butter, coconut oil, and avocado.

In an interview with PeopleTV, she explained that legumes, nuts, protein, and eggs also made their way onto her plate along with lots of veggies. She explained that it was far from deprivation. She said, "You can eat all the food you want. You can eat a big-ass porterhouse steak if you want. You just can't have the baked potato."

You can easily see all of her favorite meals on her Instagram page. She also finds inspiration from Maria Emmerich. Here's what Halle's typical day looks like:

- Breakfast – Bulletproof collagen protein or greens and beets.

- Lunch – prosciutto and arugula roll-ups or green beans and Bolognese

- Dinner – instant pot white chicken chili or arctic char with olive salsa

- Snacks – tomato tulips, chicken bone broth, or zucchini chips

The Ketogenic diet is definitely working for Halle, and it is a perfect way to help her with her diabetes.

Conclusion

Congratulations of finishing the Modern Ketogenic Diet.

Taking the first steps toward a healthy life is one of the hardest and bravest things that people can do. By choosing to try a Keto diet, you are making that step. Use the information you have learned to make the transition easier and more fulfilling. The best place to start would probably be by figuring out your macros and then going through your house and cleaning out Keto-unfriendly foods.

This won't be the easiest thing you have done in life, but it will be fulfilling. You will notice changes quickly, and if you stick to your macros, you will see the weight fall off. You can enjoy the diet. With a little creativity, you can enjoy the most delicious meals you've ever had, and you won't feel like you're missing out on anything.

Make sure that you have your goals set and have all of the foods you need to be a success. Make sure that you have plenty of fats because that will be what keeps you full. Snacks may also be a great option. Play around with your macros to figure out what works for you. The important thing is that you make this diet work for you. Now, go get started.

Finally, if you found this book useful in any way, a review on Amazon is always appreciated!

CPSIA information can be obtained
at www.ICGtesting.com
Printed in the USA
FFHW011258230919
55170690-60881FF

9 780648 562139